THE LIFE OF A
MEDICAL
OFFICER
IN WORLD WAR ONE

To the memory of Captain Harry Gordon Parker, and all those
who lost their lives in the First World War

Unarmed they bore an equal burden,
Shared each adventure undismayed.
Not less they earned the Victor's guerdon,
Not least were these in the crusade.
R.B.P., 'Hymn to the Fallen of the Royal Army Medical Corps', *1947*

THE LIFE OF A
MEDICAL OFFICER
IN WORLD WAR ONE

THE EXPERIENCES OF CAPTAIN
HARRY GORDON PARKER

LORRAINE EVANS

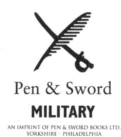

Pen & Sword
MILITARY

AN IMPRINT OF PEN & SWORD BOOKS LTD.
YORKSHIRE - PHILADELPHIA

First published in Great Britain in 2023 by
PEN AND SWORD MILITARY
An imprint of
Pen & Sword Books Limited
Yorkshire – Philadelphia

ISBN 978 1 39904 160 7

Typeset in Times New Roman 11.5/14.5 by
SJmagic DESIGN SERVICES, India.
Printed and bound in the UK by CPI Group (UK) Ltd.

Pen & Sword Books Limited incorporates the imprints of Atlas, Archaeology,
Aviation, Discovery, Family History, Fiction, History, Maritime, Military,
Military Classics, Politics, Select, Transport, True Crime, Air World, Frontline
Publishing, Leo Cooper, Remember When, Seaforth Publishing, The Praetorian
Press, Wharncliffe Local History, Wharncliffe Transport, Wharncliffe True Crime
and White Owl.

For a complete list of Pen & Sword titles please contact
PEN & SWORD BOOKS LIMITED
George House, Units 12 & 13, Beevor Street, Off Pontefract Road,
Barnsley, South Yorkshire, S71 1HN, England
E-mail: enquiries@pen-and-sword.co.uk
Website: www.pen-and-sword.co.uk

or
PEN AND SWORD BOOKS
1950 Lawrence Rd, Havertown, PA 19083, USA
E-mail: uspen-and-sword@casematepublishers.com
Website: www.penandswordbooks.com

Contents

Preface		vii
Author's Note		ix
List of Illustrations		x
List of Military Abbreviations		xiii
Acknowledgements		xv
Foreword		xvi
Introduction		xviii
Chapter 1	Wounded Belgians	1
Chapter 2	The Army	8
Chapter 3	France	18
Chapter 4	Richbourg	23
Chapter 5	Neuve Chapelle	28
Chapter 6	Dentistry	31
Chapter 7	The Somme	34
Chapter 8	A Month's Rest	38
Chapter 9	The Dreaded Fever	42
Chapter 10	France and the Third Battle of Arras	49
Chapter 11	Myself a Hospital Case	54
Chapter 12	Nieuport	59
Chapter 13	The Manchesters' Passchendaele	63
Chapter 14	Trench Feet a Crime	69
Chapter 15	The Advance – le Quesnoy	77

Chapter 16	The Last Scalp	85
Chapter 17	A Hero's End	88
Chapter 18	'La Deliverance'	92
Chapter 19	Occupation of the Rhineland	95
Chapter 20	Buel and Bonn	97
Chapter 21	'Corkey'	104
Chapter 22	Sentence of Death	110
Conclusion		116
Appendix I	Timeline of Army Medical Services (RAMC sources)	119
Appendix II	Battles on the Western Front in Flanders and France	121
Appendix III	Glossary of Place Names	126
Appendix IV	Base Hospitals on the Western Front	139
Appendix V	Classification of wounds used by British Army	143
Appendix VI	Trench Foot and Lice	145
Appendix VII	A Brief History of The Lancashire Fusiliers	149
Appendix VIII	A Brief History of The Manchester Regiment	152
Notes and References		156
Select Bibliography		158

Preface

Life of a Medical Officer in World War One delivers an intimate portrayal of life and death on the Western Front. They are the memoirs of one Captain Harry Gordon Parker, a combination of notes and jottings that offer the reader a unique first-hand account into life on the frontline for those who served in a medical capacity.

Born in Gosforth, Cumberland, on 18 September 1885, Captain Harry Gordon Parker came from a long lineage of professionals who once served in a military capacity. His great grandfather was Captain Charles Parker RN, whist his grandfather was Captain Charles Allan Parker of the Royal Marines. In Gosforth church, Cumbria, there is a large marble plaque commemorating the latter's death, who was famously killed on active service during the Crimean War (1853-56). His father was the renowned amateur antiquarian Charles Arundel Parker, famed for his writings on the Gosforth Cross, along with other ancient monuments throughout the Cumbria area, as well as a prominent medical consultant, first practising in Dumfriesshire and then afterwards in Cumbria. His mother was Agatha Smith, daughter of the celebrated Edinburgh physician Dr John Smith, dentist to Queen Victoria. Captain Harry Gordon Parker was the youngest of three sons, all of whom served during the First World War, the eldest served through the East African campaign, whilst the middle son was a commander in the Royal Navy. Having spent his formative years at Durham Boarding School, like his father before him, Harry Gordon was accepted into the University of Edinburgh to study medicine.

On 15 August 2014, at the outbreak of the First World War, Captain Harry Gordon Parker journeyed directly to the War Office in London to enlist. Successful, he initially joined the Naval Medical Service, as a Royal Navy temporary surgeon, and was sent to Southampton to work on the hospital evacuation ship the SS *St Petersburg*, later renamed *Archangel*. Somewhat disillusioned with the whole experience, he requested a transfer to the Royal Medical Army Corps. His appeal was accepted and he soon found himself transported to the front line in France. It was here, first serving with the Lancashire Fusiliers and then later as permanent Regimental Medical Officer with 2nd Manchester Regiment, that he spent the remainder of the war.

After the Armistice, Captain Harry Gordon Parker served out his remaining contract in peacetime Germany. Upon leaving the Royal Army Medical Corps, like thousands before him, Parker returned to civilian life, working as a local general medical practitioner. He died on 26 December 1969 at Park Nook, Gosforth, Seascale, Cumbria.

Author's Note

The work and experiences of the men of the Royal Army Medical Corps arguably have a profound implication for our understanding of the war. The following not only represents a faithful rendition of the account of Captain Harry Gordon Parker RAMC, but also, I hope, adds to this immense body of historical work. After much deliberation it was decided to leave the text 'as is,' rather than incorporate any modern day nuances or spelling alternatives. Any confusions or misinterpretation of events by Parker at the time have been duly noted in the Notes and References section. A supplementary historical copy, focusing on the work of the Royal Army Medical Corps and the chain of evacuation on the Western Front, has also been added to augment Parker's writings, all relevant to the original text. No personal discussion or interpretation has been added, the aim being to give the reader an informed outlook on the medical process at hand. In a similar vein, photographs from public archives have been used wherever it has been considered they might enhance the narrative landscape. Every effort has been made to contact all relevant copyright holders, to whom I am eternally grateful. However, at the end of the day I am only human, and if an error or omission has been made, I apologise most profusely. As a final word I believe it is fair to say that no active serviceman tells other than the truth as he sees it at the time of writing home or making notes when on the front line, or from any portion of the lines of communication. To such daily scribblings and jottings, we should be eternally grateful.

Lorraine Evans
Wester Ross, March 2022

Lorraine Evans can be followed at www.lorraineevans.com

List of Illustrations

Figure 1: Photograph of Captain Harry Gordon Parker, in full-dress uniform, taken at the family House, Park Nook, Gosforth, Cumbria. (Image courtesy of C. Cooper)

Figure 2: University of Edinburgh Roll of Honour, Record of Service, 1914-1918. Captain Harry Gordon Parker is listed fourth from the bottom. (National Library of Scotland. Public Domain)

Figure 3: Royal Army Medical Corps diagram of the chain of casualty evacuation. (Wellcome Collection Attribution 4.0 International CC BY 4.0)

Figure 4: Grey-wash drawing of Royal Army Medical Corps working in the trenches after a severe engagement. Fortunino Matania. (Wellcome Collection Attribution 4.0 International CC BY 4.0)

Figure 5: Postcard of Royal Army Medical Corps administering aid to the wounded. Raphael Tuck and Sons. (Wellcome Collection Attribution 4.0 International CC BY 4.0)

Figure 6: First World War Regimental Aid Post. (Wellcome Collection First World War Regimental Aid Post)

Figure 7: Medical Officer's equipment, Memorial Museum, Passchendaele. (ThruTheseLines Attribution 4.0 International CC BY 4.0)

Figure 8: Stretcher bearers lifting a casualty into a Regimental Aid Post. (National Library of Scotland. Attribution 4.0 International CC BY 4.0)

Figure 9: Plaster plaque of stretcher bearers carrying wounded soldier 1914-1920, Science Museum, London. (Wellcome Collection Attribution 4.0 International CC BY 4.0)

Figure 10: Bandaging the wounded in the field. (Wellcome Collection Attribution 4.0 International CC BY 4.0)

Figure 11: German and British wounded soldiers waiting to be evacuated, Grevillers, Bapume. (Wellcome Collection L0009184 Attribution 4.0 International CC BY 4.0)

Figure 12: Coloured charcoal drawing depicting a physician attending to a soldier in the trenches. (Wellcome Collection No. 2436i Public Domain Mark)

Figure 13: Medical Officer noting down a wounded soldier's details at a collection point. (Wellcome Collection Attribution 4.0 International CC BY 4.0)

Figure 14: Royal Army Medical Corps at Monchy dressing station, France. (Rijksmuseum, Amsterdam RP-F-F06305 CCO.1.0 Universal Public Domain Dedication)

Figure 15: Advance Dressing Station in the field, France. (Wellcome Collection Attribution 4.0 International CC BY 4.0)

Figure 16: First World War dressing station. (Wellcome Collection No L0009298 Attribution 4.0 International CC BY 4.0)

Figure 17: First aid on the battlefield at Advance Dressing Station on the Somme front line. (Wellcome Collection Attribution 4.0 International CC BY 4.0)

Figure 18: Diorama of Western Front dressing station. Science Museum, London. (Wellcome Collection Attribution 4.0 International CC BY 4.0)

Figure 19: Casualty Clearing Station on the Western Front. (National Library of Scotland Attribution 4.0 International CC BY 4.0)

Figure 20: Remains of Hospital St Jean, Arras after heavy shelling by the Germans. (CC BY 4.0 Public Domain)

Figure 21: Grey-wash drawing of horse ambulance at Ypres by Sir D. Lindsay. (Wellcome Collection Attribution 4.0 International CC BY 4.0)

Figure 22: Mock-up of First World War horse-drawn ambulance. Royal Logistic Corps Museum. G. Cornelius. (Attribution 4.0 International CC BY 4.0)

Figure 23: Grey-wash drawing of Red Cross ambulance train loading up the wounded at a Casualty Clearing Station. D. Lindsay. (Wellcome Collection Attribution 4.0 International CC BY 4.0)

Figure 24: First World War ambulance train. (Wellcome Collection Attribution 4.0 International CC BY 4.0)

Figure 25: First World War motor ambulance. (Wellcome Collection Attribution 4.0 International CC BY 4.0)

Figure 26: Patients carried aboard a hospital barge on the Western Front. (Dutch National Archives. CCC 1.0 Public Domain Dedication)

Figure 27: Wounded being carried from a British hospital ship. (Wellcome Collection Attribution 4.0 International CC BY 4.0)

Figure 28: Map of the Battle of the Somme 1916. (GiroUS Attribution 4.0 International CC BY 3.0)

Figure 29: Soldiers carrying duckboards across the mud-filled landscape of Passchendaele by W. Rider. (Image Library and Archives, Canada. Public Domain Mark)

Figure 30: Trench feet Image No. 155 King George Military Hospital. (Wellcome Collection CMACRAMC 760/L0025834 Attribution 4.0 International CC BY 4.0)

Figure 31: Osbourne House, Queen Victoria's family retreat, Isle of Wight. Used as a convalescent home for military officers during the First World War. (Sulcasmo Attribution 4.0 International CC BY 4.0)

Figure 32: Commemoration dedicated to the Royal Army Medical Corps, Westminster Abbey. (Author's photograph)

List of Military Abbreviations

ADGMS	Assistant Director General of Medical Services
ADMS	Assistant Director of Medical Services
AFA	Advance Field Ambulance
ASC	Army Service Corps
BEF	British Expeditionary Force
BHQ	Battalion Headquarters
BMJ	*British Medical Journal*
CCS	Casualty Clearing Station
CSF	Comprehensive Soldier Fitness
CO	Commanding Officer
CSM	Company Sergeant Major
DMS	Director of Medical Services
DDMS	Deputy Director of Medical Services
DORA	Defence of the Realm Act
DSM	Distinguished Service Medal
DLI	Durham Light Infantry
FA	Field Ambulance
HLI	Highland Light Infantry
ICT	Inflammation Connection Tissue
KC	Knight Commander

LF	Lancashire Fusiliers
MO	Medical Officer
MR	Manchester Regiment
NCO	Non-Commissioned Officer
OC	Officer Commanding
PMO	Principal Medical Officer
PUO	Pyrexia of Unknown Origin
QM	Quartermaster
RAMC	Royal Army Medical Corps
RAP	Regimental Aid Post
RE	Royal Engineers
RMO	Regimental Medical Officer
RNMS	Royal Naval Medical Service
RTO	Railway Transport Officer
SMO	Senior Medical Officer
TMB	Travelling Medical Board
VAD	Voluntary Aid Detachment
VC	Victoria Cross
WAAC	Women's Auxiliary Army Corps
YSB	Young Soldiers Battalion

Acknowledgements

I would like to express my gratitude to the following people for their invaluable support and assistance: to my publishers Pen and Sword, in particular to my Commissioning Editor Jonathan Wright and Publishing Assistant Charlotte Mitchell; to my Copy Editor, esteemed Military Historian Richard Doherty; Kate Bohdanowicz for her advice and efforts in pushing the manuscript forward; Thomas Watson and Lou Labelle for being my support network during the writing of this book; to the staff at The National Archives, The Imperial War Museum, the Wellcome Collection, the National Library of Scotland, the Irish Guards, the Manchester Regiment and Lancashire Fusiliers for their advice and archival/image research; Dr John Apres; and finally members of the Cooper family. I would also like to extend my appreciation to those on certain media platforms who have offered their support and knowledge unquestionably.

Foreword

Captain Harry G. Parker RAMC

At the beginning of the war, a certain famous daily paper loudly proclaimed that there would be 'better doctoring after the war', as the result of the experience gained. It did not take much imagination or foresight to realise that, for the ordinary doctor, experience useful in civil life would be practically nil, except at the base hospitals. But even at the base this hope proved to be illusionary. Cases when fit to travel were transferred to England, and the surgeons were unable to follow them up and know the results of their work. One surgeon told me that he had taken much trouble to ascertain the whereabouts of certain of his patients in England and had written imploring letters begging just a little information as to the progress of this or that case, but that he had never had one single reply to any of the communications.

Surgically, two things stood out as a result of the war on the Western Front. A great advance in the surgery of the lung, and much experience gained in regard to infected (septic) fractures of the larger bones. The Medical Services were called upon for the first time to deal with casualties resulting from gas and evolved no effective treatment for the severer cases. Amidst so much sepsis certain 'laissez-faire' showed itself in a slackening of the normal aseptic regime. Red tape flourished, however, as in other branches of the Service.

A Naval MO was not allowed to operate until he became a Fleet Surgeon. It took about twenty years to attain Fleet Surgeon rank, by which time a surgeon's hand had lost any original cunning that it may have possessed. I saw one of these Fleet Surgeons operate for removal of the appendix. It was heart-breaking to watch him, for he took half an hour to open the abdomen – time enough to complete the average operation of appendectomy. But it was clear that he might have been a good surgeon, had he been allowed to operate during the past fifteen years. The amount of confidence that the Admiralty had in their naval surgeons was demonstrated by the fact that they appointed two civilian specialists to the hospital at a salary of £5,000 a year each to perform operations. These two surgeons spent most of their time walking round the hospital looking for someone to operate on.

In the first week of the war I tried hard to enlist, and at the War Office found myself at the tail of a large crowd who stood on some steps running along the side of the building. In the middle of the crowd was an alley-way lined by police, leading up to the door. I enquired of a mounted policeman as to where I should go to enlist as a civil surgeon. He directed me to another officer. I started to advance towards this individual. The crowd thought that I was getting somewhere, out of my turn, and made an ugly rush, sweeping aside the line of police. Next moment the mounted police were backing their horses into the crowd. I made myself scarce and tried the front door, with the result that I was hustled out of the War Office and ordered to move on. I was very much afraid of 'missing' the war altogether and eventually managed to get into the Navy. They sent me to Devonport.

Here there were a score of more temporary MOs in addition to the normal staff, and the hospital was practically empty in readiness for the big naval battle that was daily expected. Rounds, however, had to be performed religiously at stated hours. You marched along the corridor and halted at the first flight of stairs. As you reached the foot of the stair a sick berth steward would appear at the top. 'No. 4 all correct?' you shouted. 'No. 4 all correct sir,' came the reply, and you passed on to the next stairway. The thing was a farce. This enforced idleness was very galling to anyone accustomed to the busy life of a civil hospital, and in a short time I paraded before the Surgeon-Admiral and asked to be sent to sea. 'Why, my boy,' said that fine-looking man, 'you've only been there five minutes. Content yourself.' This perforce I tried to do.

What struck one most about the Naval Medical Service was the cordial dislike which all officers seemed to have for their immediate superiors. It was not a contented service by any means, and many regulations were better in theory than in practice.

Introduction

In October 1854 *The Times* newspaper ran a series of articles by Thomas Chenery, their correspondent in Constantinople, condemning the provision of medical care for British soldiers serving in the Crimean War (1853-6). Observing a marked absence of surgeons and nurses, together with lack of medical supplies, Chenery noted that 'The worn-out pensioners who were brought out as an ambulance corps are totally useless, and not only are surgeons not to be had, but there are no dresser or nurses to carry out the surgeon's directions and attend on the sick during intervals between his visits'. Added to this debacle was the lack of status afforded to the medical profession in general. As Ian Whitehead states in *Doctors in the Great War*, medical officers at this time were not regarded as fellow officers, merely 'camp followers,' a state of affairs that, regrettably, would persist. They had no authority over regimental troops, their pay fell well below that of other officers and they often had to meet expenses related to their medical duties out of their own pockets. Moreover, Whitehead notes that regardless of acts of gallantry performed by medical officers in the Crimean War, military honours had largely been denied them. Only three received the Victoria Cross, which is more than during the Second World War.

While medical support to the armed forces can be traced back to at least the seventeenth century (see Appendix I), the fiasco of the Crimean War eventually gave rise to a series of governmental enquiries, which in turn led to the creation, in 1855, of a Medical Staff Corps of men who were allocated solely to hospital work. In 1898, by Royal Warrant, the Medical Staff Corps merged with The Army Medical Department, an officers-only corps formed in 1873, to create the Royal Army Medical Corps. Their first significant field of operation would arise one year later, during the Second Anglo-Boer War (1899-1902), which historian

Dr Jessica Myers argues played a significant role in the development of military medical services in Britain. Whereas John Blair goes one step further and suggests that 'in this South African ... conflict, the Royal Army Medical Corps made its own transition from an irregularly organised, civilian-orientated service of the 19th century to the fully organised professional Corps of the Army of the 20th.' What is generally agreed is that the experiences gained throughout this conflict would shape the Royal Army Medical Corps as it took to the field in France in 1914. At the outbreak of the First World War, just sixteen years after its formation, there were 9,000 warrant officers and men of the RAMC; this grew to 113,000 by 1918.

The role of an RAMC Medical Officer (MO) during the First World War was a varied, albeit precarious, one. Each fighting unit would have their own doctor, a Regimental Medical Officer (RMO) who came under the Commanding Officer (CO) of that particular unit. Their responsibilities not only related to the care and welfare of the sick and wounded, but equally to matters of sanitation, which extended to the supply of water and preparation of food. In the early years of the war, as Whitehead notes, there was definitely some confusion and uncertainty with regards to their exact duties. Many MOs were unclear as to exactly how much risk they were expected to take whilst on duty, resulting in many RMOs leaving the relative safety of their RAP and rushing forward to treat their wounded colleagues:

> Doc here was always in the thick of it. By rights he should have been back at the RAP waiting for casualties to be brought back. But not him, he was right up there in the attack, going over the top with the men, attending to them as they got wounded.
>
> Officer of the Wiltshire Regiment,
> describing their RMO.

Alarmingly, by 1917, the death rate among RMOs and their orderlies was reportedly as high as forty per 1,000 per month. Despite this figure and considering the large numbers of casualties per day, reaching on average somewhere between 15,000 to 20,000, it has been documented that, on the Western Front alone, the wounded that returned to the firing line due to the medical attention they received represented a manpower saving of 1,600,000. Such a feat would have been impossible without a high degree of organisation. It had been realised very early on in the war that a man's chance of survival depended on how quickly his injuries could be treated. As a result of those observations, a new scheme was swiftly implemented, known as the Chain of Evacuation (Figure 3). Each stage of the operation had its own agenda, but the goal was the same for all: to treat the wounded and return them back to the frontline as soon as possible.

The Casualty Evacuation Line

Regimental Aid Posts

The initial journey from the battlefield to a medical post for a wounded soldier on the Western Front varied depending on the injuries sustained. More often than not, the first port of call would be a Regimental Aid Post (RAP), which was situated in or close to the frontline position. It was the Regimental Medical Officer's (RMO) responsibility to establish an Aid Post as near to the firing line as was deemed safe. Here a casualty would have his first encounter with a trained medical professional, namely the RMO, assisted by a series of orderlies and trained stretcher-bearers. The RMO would check that the wounds were clean, oversee the strapping of any damaged and/or fractured limbs and, on rare occasions, carry out any necessary emergency amputations. As the RAP was the first point of call on the front line, prevention of shock was also a primary concern. In essence, the responsibility of the MO was to ensure that the casualty was in a fit state to be moved along the line of evacuation.

The MO was also responsible for completing a full field medical card for each patient, fixing it firmly about their person. This card included the soldier's name, rank, unit and diagnosis and was meant to provide a consecutive record of the patient's condition and treatment in his passage through the field ambulance, casualty clearing stations and the hospitals on the lines of communication. Once the necessary details were collected, the patient would then be taken from the RAP to a designated collecting area to be picked up by stretcher-bearers of the field ambulance.

The RAP would move forward in line with the conflict, so it needed to be able to re-deploy at a moment's notice. They had no holding capacity for the wounded and, at first, were typically located in a dugout, a communication trench, a ruined house or, at times, even in a deep shell hole. They were badly lit, had limited space and, on many occasions, prone to flooding. As a result, any significant examination of a patient was extremely challenging. Nonetheless, even this small amount of shelter could offer crucial protection from enemy shelling. By 1917 the typical RAP had evolved somewhat from its crude beginnings and now resembled a '(cross-shaped) heavily propped and timbered series of wide passages, with a central compartment wide enough to allow stretchers to pass.' Bunks were built into the walls to accommodate the wounded, whilst separate compartments were constructed for the MO and his staff. On the battlefield a yellow flag was erected, often adjacent to a RAP, so that those wounded in no man's land could find it. When under pressure, the RMO could be further assisted with members from a Field Ambulance upon request.

Supplies were provided by the aforementioned Field Ambulance and normally consisted of a primus stove and a Beatrice stove, along with an acetylene lamp together with an assortment of medical necessities. In 1914 the basic MO's drug box included: 'Phenacetin for headaches, Adrenaline in injectable form.... Dover's powders for colds, Bismuth salicylate for the stomach, cough medicine, quinine sulphate and opium tablets to be made into a lotion as an application for sprains ... . and for the doctor to administer safely morphine sulphate,' as well as an anti-tetanus serum, assorted bandages, blankets, Boric ointment, cotton wool, first field dressings and so on. There were also a hamper containing comforts such as brandy, cocoa, Bovril, oxo and biscuits. The RMO would be equipped with a horse for his personal use, a Maltese cart, in essence a two-wheeled cart suitable for transporting a prone patient, and, if very fortunate, he might also have access to a light motor van or a small motor-car.

Field Ambulance

The Field Ambulance (FA) was not a vehicle, but a mobile medical unit comprising ten officers and 224 men when at full strength. It consisted of three previously independent entities, namely the bearer division (previously working as bearer companies), which contained eighteen stretcher squads, each of six men; the tent division (previously working as field hospitals), which had doctors, nine MOs and one dental officer, together with a quartermaster of stores, batmen, clerks, cooks, dispensers and nursing orderlies, whilst the transport division (Army Service Corps), had sixty men all told. All three bodies made up the medical support for a singular infantry brigade, with each brigade encompassing three to four battalions respectively. The Field Ambulance was further divided into A, B and C sections, with each section quite capable of carrying out independent action. The field ambulance headquarters always formed part of A Section.

In the trenches its role was similar to a modern-day emergency ambulance service, collecting the wounded from a designated RAP and transporting them down the chain of evacuation to an appropriate treatment centre. This could be within the confines of the tent division, where the wounded would often receive some primary care, after which they would return to their unit, or be evacuated down the line to an Advanced Dressing Station (ADS). When away from the front line the role of the Field Ambulance was to keep the men in tip-top fighting condition, which would comprise the formation of divisional rest stations (DRS) and/or communal bathing stations.

A brief mention should also be made of the cavalry field ambulance, which was the same as the standard Field Ambulance, the only difference being that it was smaller and more mobile. It consisted of six RAMC officers and seventy other ranks. There were four Field Ambulances per cavalry division, each divided into both A and B Sections.

> The usual procedure in action is that the ambulance is
> divided into tent and bearer sections, the former of which
> establish a temporary hospital of fifty beds some five miles
> behind the firing line. The bearer section goes forward and
> gets into touch with the regiment attached RAMC Officer
> at this regimental aid post when the cavalry are engaged
> in reconnaissance. From the aid post they will move cases
> in light wagons to the temporary hospital ... . Professional
> work for officers consists of emergency operations and quick
> evacuation of wounded to the lines of communication. It does

not burden itself with chronic cases, as it is a highly mobile force and must be ready to move forward at the shortest possible notice in conjunction with the cavalry brigade.

Major H. Norman Barnett RAMC
The Work of a Cavalry Field Ambulance

Advanced Dressing Station

The Advance Dressing Station (ADS) was the first line of administration for the RAMC, whereby records of admissions and discharge were noted together with engagement documentation on the front line. Each ADS comprised three officers, one designated officer commanding, and fifty-three other ranks. Thirty-six privates would be employed as stretcher-bearers, the others as clerks, dressers and cooks. Personnel numbers could be increased if the station became overwhelmed with casualties. Each ADS was duly equipped with the necessary items such as stretchers, flags for marking routes and notice boards, as well as much-needed medical paraphernalia, including field bandages, anti-tetanus serum, iodine, plasters and splints for leg and back injuries. Surgery was not undertaken at the ADS unless it was deemed absolutely necessary. They were simply an intermediate stop-off point to assess the patient. Having received a casualty from an RAP, basic medical treatment, such as checking dressings, would be administered before the patient would be transferred onwards. Those deemed urgent cases would be transferred to the Main Dressing Station (MDS), whilst those who were not would be conveyed directly to a Casualty Clearing Station (CCS). At times it would be impossible to site an ADS close to the front line, predominantly due to unsuitable topography caused by heavy shelling. Under such circumstances the Field Ambulance would set up intermediate posts, known as bearer relay posts (BRP), roughly sited every half mile between the RAP, FA and ADS, thus making it easier for stretcher-bearers to carry their loads across the difficult terrain. There were no medical facilities at these posts; they merely existed to enable the stretcher-bearers to pass the casualty to the next set of stretcher-bearers.

Main Dressing Station

Main Dressing Stations (MDS) were formed by the headquarters of the field ambulance, namely Section A. They consisted of a commanding officer, two medical officers, a dental officer, a quartermaster and fifty-nine other RAMC ranks, along with one Army Service Corps officer, and forty-four other ranks. The MDS was sited further away from the firing line than an ADS, ideally approximately one mile back, but this was rarely achieved on the Western Front, due to the ever-changing landscape. In an ideal situation they needed to be located between the ADS and a casualty clearing station, if possible, in a large building with existing running water, light and heating. If this was unobtainable, then approximately nine tents were used, with one reserved as an operating room. As the station was further back from the firing line, it was better equipped to perform urgent operations, having access to all-important oxygen apparatus, collapsible trestles and operating lights.

Bar officers' accommodation, a cookhouse, stores and designated mortuary, each MDS was divided into six sections: 1) Receiving Section provided hot drinks and food; 2) Recording Section where clerks recorded the patient's information from his field medical card; 3) Resuscitation Section for warming and receiving those suffering from shock of the effects of haemorrhage; 4) Dressing Station where dressings were applied, and any urgent medical treatment administered; 5) Gas Section to keep gas victims away from other patients and, finally, 6) Evacuation Section where the patients awaited evacuation.

Walking Wounded Collection Point (WWCP)

If, during a major offensive, and it was deemed that the ADS would become overcrowded, a walking wounded collection point (WWCP) would be created at a location between the ADS and MDS, at a point which provided easy access from the front line, and close to the stretcher-bearers' route. Staffed predominantly from field ambulance personnel, there were no specific arrangements of equipment, bar a reception section, a recording section and a dressing station. No operations or complicated medical assistance were provided. It was simply an intermediate post to determine where the patient should be transferred next.

Casualty Clearing Station

Casualty Clearing Stations (CCS) were pivotal to the whole practice of evacuating the wounded away from the front. Until early 1915 they were known simply as clearing stations, and their role would evolve considerably throughout the war. Located farther back from the front line than RAPs and FAs, they were sited on or near railway lines to facilitate the movement of casualties from the battlefield to the hospitals. They were manned by troops from the RAMC, the Army Service Corps and personnel from the Royal Engineers. Under normal circumstances CCS personnel would include eight MOs, one quartermaster, seven nurse from the Queen Alexandra's Imperial Military Nursing Service and seventy-seven other ranks working in various departments such as nursing orderlies, theatre orderlies, cooks etc. Often a dentist and/or pathologist was attached to the station, as well as a chaplain, electricians and various lorry/ambulance drivers. Such numbers, though, were woefully inadequate for wartime and, more often than not, the personnel would be increased to include a specialised 'surgical team.' This comprised a surgeon, an anaesthetist, a theatre sister, two theatre orderlies, four stretcher-bearers and a batman. The latter were usually brought in from base hospitals or from other CCSs that were not currently engaged in active operations.

> It was not advisable to make elaborate arrangements for serious surgical operations on patients within the zone of ordinary shell-fire. Therefore, as a routine, only such operations as are absolutely necessary should be performed in units in front of the casualty clearing stations. Operations for haemorrhage which threatens life, and those for the removal of hopelessly smashed limbs ate the only ones ought to be done.
>
> *The early Treatment of War Wounds*,
> Colonel H.M.W. Gray

CCSs were large, static, well-equipped medical facilities, usually located in a large building, if available, or a series of tented camps and huts. Customarily, there was one CCS per division but, during a major offensive, this number would increase tenfold. By September 1916, every CCS was divided into a heavy and light section. The light section was highly mobile in practice and could move back and forth with the troops on the front line. It was also used to set up specialist epicentres, specifically advance operating centres and abdominal hospitals. Usually working in twos or threes, this meant manpower could be spread evenly throughout the field of conflict depending on demand. When one CCS was closed to treat the wounded brought in by train or ambulance, the other would be preparing itself to receive new casualties. When the second one reached its capacity, the first station would be empty and available to receive new casualties. Thus, the cycle continued. If a third station was working in rotation, it would either be treating the sick, or could evacuate at a moment's notice to tend to emergencies. On average each CCS took around 150-200 wounded before they would close their doors to new arrivals. This number would significantly increase by 1917 to between 800 to 1,200 sick and wounded. Typically, a CCS was not a place for long-term convalescence.

The role of the CCS evolved significantly as the war forged ahead, and the CCS of 1918 was unrecognisable from its establishment in 1914. In fact, with equipment still being transported to the front-line areas in 1914, the stations never really became fully functioning units until the year 1915. With an influx of urgent cases, such as abdominal injuries and gangrene, to attend to, in that same year the Director General of Medical Services approved the movement of surgical services in the CCS, whereby the most serious wounds were now sent directly to a CCS, bypassing other sections on the front line. Serious operations, such as limb amputations, could be performed, together with specialist medical units to treat infectious diseases, such as VD, trench foot, nervous disorders, and brain injuries. Incoming casualties were first assessed and divided into three categories: non-serious cases – to be returned to duty after rest and recuperation; serious cases but fit to travel – to be immediately evacuated back to a base hospital and serious cases in urgent need of immediate treatment. More often than not, the casualty would be moved to a base hospital (BH). The wounded were provided with food and rest, the main objective being to provide necessary treatment and move them out as quickly as possible. In fact, the CCS was looked upon by many of the men as their first real haven of rest. The majority of evacuated casualties came away from the CCS by rail, although motor ambulances and canal barges were also in operation. In 1916, on the Western Front alone, 734,000 wounded men were evacuated from CCSs by train and another 17,000 by inland water transport. That same year efforts were made to bring the CCS even closer to the front line, in order to try and reduce deaths amongst the most severely injured men, who might bleed to death whilst awaiting transport.

By 1917, records show that more operations were performed at a CCS than at a base hospital, with individual CCSs allocated to treat specific injuries, including measures to deal with mustard gas, used by the Germans for a time during that year. Another improvement was the training of nursing sisters in the provision of anaesthetics, which naturally freed up a large number of MOs for other duties. However, by 1918, it was deemed unsuitable to have the CCSs so close to the front line, where artillery shelling from enemy action was ever present. They were subsequently moved back. Today, the location of CCSs along the Western Front can often be determined from the cluster of cemeteries that once encircled them.

Base Hospitals

The concluding phase of the casualty evacuation chain, on the Western Front, was a base hospital, which was sited further back from the front line than a CCS. There were two types, known as stationary and general hospitals and, once admitted, a wounded soldier stood a reasonable chance of survival. They needed to be close to a railway line, in order for casualties to arrive, but also near a port where men could be evacuated for treatment in Britain. Manned once more by troops from the RAMC, together with Army Service Corps and personnel from the Royal Engineers, they were generally located near the coast, in large buildings, often within seaside hotels. The stationary hospital, two per division, could hold approximately 400 casualties at one time, whereas a general hospital could hold many more, around 1,040 patients. This figure increased significantly in 1917 to as many as 2,500 beds. It was rare for such large establishments to move with the fighting, until 1918 where some hospitals moved into the Rhine bridgehead in Germany. Many were still active in France well into 1919 (see Appendix IV).

Transport of the Wounded

Understandably, the effectiveness of the casualty evacuation system was determined by how quickly the patient could be transferred to the next medical station down the line and was dependent of three overriding factors: time – how rapidly a casualty can get to recognised medical personnel + how quickly wounds become infected; space – is there room to set up a medical facility close-by + topography; transport – what type of equipment can be used and is it readily available. Here follows a brief overview of the transportation methods typically employed.

Horse Drawn Transport

According to the *Royal Army Medical Corps Training Manual, 1911*, Guideline No.329, 'in every country, where the roads permit of wheeled ambulance transport, vehicles of varying design, drawn by horses, ponies, mules or oxen, form the chief means of transporting the sick and wounded.' This viewpoint was still acknowledged at the outbreak of the First World War, when the Army required thousands of civilian horses to serve alongside its armed forces. Together with their drivers, horse-drawn ambulances remained in service throughout the war and, by 1917, the Army had employed over 368,000 horses on the Western Front. They were far more suited to the heavy-shelled landscape than motor transport, one of many examples is the clearing of the wounded at Pozieres, who had been brought down by horse trolley from the fighting at Courcelette in 1916. That is not to say that the use of the horse did not present a challenge. There was a constant need for sufficient food and water supplies, combined with the difficulty of dealing with the sheer scale of corpses that could not be buried at one time. Along the position of the Aisne, for instance, the bodies of whole teams of horses lay piled up, struck down by shell-fire and left to rot. The British troops did their best in most cases of this kind, but it was impossible to bury all the carcasses, and thus the work of the RAMC was rendered doubly hard with regards to sanitation, as there was a danger of infection to troops for miles around.

Different types of horse were suited to different military roles. Riding horses were naturally deployed to the cavalry section and were used as officers' mounts. Small but strong multi-purpose horses and ponies were ideally suited to carrying heavy shells and ammunition. Draught horses, which were used to pulling buses back in Britain, were not only good for hauling heavy artillery guns and supplies, but also ideally built for the pulling of ambulance wagons, especially across badly shell-damaged roads. The particulars of each horse-drawn wagon would evolve as the war progressed, with the British Army preferring, Mark V*, Mark VI and Mark I (Light) styles. Each could carry at least four sick or wounded passengers on stretchers, two on the floor and two on the rails, which folded down on the forward seats, or twelve sitting patients, six on each side. A particular favourite of the RAMC, which formed part of the medical equipment of a battalion, was the Maltese Cart, a small two-wheeled cart, with accompanying gears, which could easily be hauled by horse, pony, mule or men.

Other Wheeled Transport

One of the developments of the First World War that still shapes healthcare today is the 'motorised ambulance.' When British troops first landed in France, in August 1914, some of the earliest casualties were still experiencing agonising bone-jolting journeys by horse-drawn wagons, to various evacuation centres. The Director General of the Army Medical Services, Sir Alfred Keogh, petitioned repeatedly for the supply of motorised vehicles, but his protestations, alas, fell on death ears. In his opinion a motor vehicle offered a number of advantages for evacuating the wounded, among them the ability to stop quickly, the capacity for operating in all weathers, fast refuelling, and reliance on gasoline rather than grazing pasture and heavy-to-transport feed, albeit on the Western Front they were not always best suited for the terrain. With both political and public criticism growing, on 12 September 1914, a small meeting was held at the Royal Automobile Club at which a few members offered to place themselves and their cars at the disposal of the Red Cross. The following month, in October 1914, *The Times* newspaper made a nationwide appeal for ambulance funds, raising enough money for the purchase and outfitting of 512 vehicles in three weeks. Finally, by the end of 1914, 'the formation of motor ambulance convoys, in proportion to the number of the divisions in the field' had become definitely authorised, and the War Office 'had prepared and despatched as many as 324 motor ambulance cars to France'. By the end of January 1915, more than 1,000 ambulances and motor vehicles of all kinds had been shipped, including a large quantity donated by various charities, such as the Red Cross and the Order of St John. In fact, the Red Cross established their very own motor ambulance department, which sent a total of 3,446 motor vehicles, including 2,171 motor ambulances, to various destinations throughout the war. By the end of 1918, eighteen complete motor ambulance convoys were on active duty overseas.

Ambulance Trains

The use of available railway networks provided the military authorities with an enormous logistical capacity to support forces in the field, including the transport of weapons and manpower. Ambulance trains thus became a fundamental part of the medical evacuation process during the First World War and successfully carried millions of sick and injured soldiers to safety. They were used at various stages along the chain of casualty evacuation, from the front line to the stationary hospitals behind. Their presence in the theatre of war, however, was not down to pure chance; they had been conceived many years beforehand. In the time leading up to 1914, in expectation of a much anticipated Europe-wide conflict, the British government had already begun secretly making plans for war. As part of this strategy, the government summoned a number of privately-owned companies, namely the Railway Executive Committee, to discuss not only how to keep the railways operational during the war, but also to debate the pros and cons behind a fully-operational fleet of ambulance trains, comprising wards, pharmacies, emergency operating rooms etc. into the confines of a train. Secret drawings were sent out to railway companies across the country so that, when war was eventually declared on 4 August 1914, the railway industry was already prepared. The first ambulance train arrived in Southampton twenty days later.

Initially the rail companies focused their attention on ambulance trains for British use only, picking up the sick and injured from various designated coastal docking areas, such as Southampton and Dover, and transporting them to hospital. It is estimated that during the course of the war the port of Dover handled a staggering 1,260,000 casualties, equating to almost 8,000 trainloads of patients. But, with the French sustaining heavy losses in manpower and rolling stock, it quickly became apparent that they could no longer supply adequate transport for the evacuation of both French and British casualties. As such, in December 1914 the Railway Executive Committee was ordered to build a fleet of continental ambulance trains to be used in France. By 1918, the railway companies had built twenty ambulance trains for use in Britain, and thirty-one for the continent.

Operation of the ambulance trains was the responsibility of the RAMC, with an RAMC major in charge of each train. They were specifically designed to be easy to clean, as a sterile environment was important to its operation. Each train could carry 500 passengers, many in critical condition, together with up to fifty staff, the majority being orderlies. The wounded were often transferred to the train while still in full uniform caked with mud and blood. MOs were responsible for checking each soldier onto the train and deciding his course of treatment. There would usually be three medical officers onboard, and two to three nurses. Each train also had chefs working in a specially designed kitchen carriage to keep everyone fed. Specific trains were adapted to meet the needs of various military organisations. For example, Naval ambulance trains were built to slightly different specifications; they had 'cots' instead of bunks so that the wounded could be transferred straight from the ship to the train without the need of a stretcher. With so many sick and injured confined into one space, naturally the working environment onboard was extremely difficult, with emergency operations performed despite the movement of the train, the cramped conditions and poor lighting. The staff were also at risk from infectious disease, lice, or being shelled by enemy fire. Despite this, many staff lived on ambulance trains throughout the war; they had their own quarters, baths and showers and some even had the luxury of heating. On the other hand, for the wounded travelling on an ambulance train could be a miserable affair; the small bunks provided were suffocating and those with broken bones felt every jolt of the carriage on the tracks. Many journeys were very long, for example travelling from Braisne to Rouen would take at least two and a half days.

The principal destination for ambulance trains abroad was a six-hectare strip of land near the French town of Étaples, overlooking the Canache estuary. This was the site of the largest military field hospital complex in France. The chain of evacuation would go as follows: light railways were used to transport the wounded to a CCS, whence another ambulance train would then move the men from the CCS to a base hospital, and from there to an evacuation port. During times of heavy conflict, many ambulance trains would come under increasing pressure to exceed the number of patients they were authorised to carry. For example, during the Battle of the Somme, Train Number 29, built by the Lancashire and Yorkshire Railway, was authorised to carry 370 patients but carried 761 on 2 July alone. Furthermore, in the first four days of the fighting (1-4 July), ambulance trains made a staggering sixty-three journeys with 33,392 men transported from railheads to bases along the coast of France. The swift evacuation of soldiers to Britain would not have been possible without these trains.

Ambulance Barges

If specially-fitted ambulance trains were not available, in some circumstances casualties would be transported via a hospital barge. Although the journey was slow, unlike a hospital train it was smooth, allowing the wounded to enjoy a certain degree of rest and recuperation. Extending to approximately seventy feet in length, and with a capacity to hold between sixteen to twenty-four prone wounded, plus twenty or more sitting patients, many were converted into travelling hospitals throughout the war. The holds were transformed into thirty-bed hospital wards, plus nurses' accommodation, and were heated by two stoves and electric lighting, which had to be turned off at night so as not to become an easy target for German fighter pilots. On the exterior, each barge would be painted grey with a large red cross on each side, together with flag poles flying a red cross, signifying they were carrying wounded soldiers.

Unlike ambulance trains, the initial motivation for their design emanated from private industry and charitable donations rather than a British government enterprise, as shown by this advertisement which appeared in a number of national newspapers from 24 to 28 December 1914:

FLOATING HOSPITALS. WATER AMBULANCES FOR BRITISH AND FRENCH TROOPS.

A small committee, of which Mr J.A. Grant, MP for the Egremont Division of Cumberland, is chairman, has been formed for the purpose of fitting out water ambulances to be used on the French and Belgian waterways. Barges are to be converted into floating hospitals. It has been found possible by this means to convey the sick and wounded from the front to a port of embarkation without suffering the agonising pains consequent upon the jolting of ambulance wagons. The scheme has the approval of Sir Arthur Sloggett, Surgeon-General at the front, and Mr Douglas Hall MP, who has already demonstrated its practicability, is leaving shortly for the front to initiate the scheme. The barges when converted will be staffed by surgeons and nurses under the control of the Royal Army Medical Corps, while voluntary assistance has been obtained which will avoid all waste money in administering the fund. Offices have been opened at 27a, St James's Street, London, where contributions will be received. Cheques should made payable to the British Water Ambulance Fund, and crossed Union of London and Smith's Bank.

The fund raised enough money to fit out four barges, which began production on the riverways of northern France, sailing on the River Seine between Paris and Rouen. Operational management was eventually taken over by the War Office, and the four barges became collectively known as Number 1 Ambulance Barge Flotilla. Each barge was manned by a non-commissioned officer, two men from the Royal Engineers Inland Waterways department, with the medical staff provided by the RAMC and the female nursing services. By the time the flotilla disbanded in November 1915, it had carried 5,230 casualties.

Before the order was given to demobilise the flotilla, in early 1915 the Surgeon General, W.G. MacPherson, DMS, suggested that three canal barges could be outfitted for use in the segregation and treatment of infectious cases. Approval was given for the proposal on 19 March 1915 and the first barge went into service only a month later, on 18 April. Five more were to follow. They were subsequently named Number 2 Ambulance Barge Flotilla. The war diary of 2 Ambulance Flotilla records that it remained in approximately the same area of operations throughout the rest of the war, with barges working in the area of Béthune, Avelette, Merville, Isberques, Aire-sur-la-Lys, Estaires, Arques, Saint-Omer and Calais. This was soon followed by Number 3 Ambulance Barge Flotilla, which entered into the fray on 17 July 1915. Led by Barge 140, which was manned by twenty troops from twenty individual Field Ambulances, it began working along the river Somme route as far as Corbie, until the end of the year when it relocated its base farther along the Somme to Chipilly. Number 4 Ambulance Barge Flotilla, also manned by twenty troops from twenty FAs, came into operation on 11 October 2015 and worked the same river and canal network as its predecessors until 1917 when it moved further north to the Dunkirk and Adinkerke areas to support the Allied forces on the Belgian coast. During July 2016 Number 3 and Number 4 units began to operate under a single command with barges working in pairs; a single MO was attached to each pair. They continued to work the Somme route, briefly advancing their base to Peronne in July 1917. The final flotilla, Number 5, came into existence at Saint-Omer on 10 July 1916 and followed the same northern canal and river network as those barges that came before. By the end of the war, more than 70,000 wounded personnel had been carried to safety from the front line by these barges.

Hospital Ships

According to Lyn MacDonald in *The Roses of No Man's Land*, around 2,261,502 wounded men were returned to the UK from the trenches of France and Flanders via hospital ships. Although their use to nurse and transport wounded personnel was not exclusive to the First World War, during both the previous Crimean and Boer wars many passenger vessels were used for transport, both to and from the front lines. Throughout the 1914-1918 conflict the Royal Navy operated a total of ninety-two hospital ships, bringing together a mixture of large passenger liners, such as the imposing RMS *Aquitania* and HMHS *Britannic*, believed to have been the largest hospital ship of the First World War, to smaller commuter and packet-type vessels, which once regularly crossed the English Channel/ North Sea. When war initially broke out, the rules of engagement clearly forbade any shelling or attack on field hospitals. This set of laws applied to hospital ships too. However, to prevent becoming a target in the first instance, ships had to adhere to a set of regulations laid down by the Hague Convention X in 1907. Entitled 'Convention for the adaptation to maritime war of the principles of the Geneva Convention,' they read as follows:

- Ship must be clearly marked and lighted as a hospital ship, including the application of white hulls, green stripes and red crosses
- Ship must give medical assistance to wounded personnel of all nationalities
- Ship must not be used for any military purpose
- Ship must not interfere with or hamper enemy combatant vessels
- Belligerents, as designated by the Hague Convention X, can search any hospital ship to investigate violations of the above restrictions
- Belligerents will establish the location of a hospital ship

Regardless of being painted in the colours deemed necessary by the Hague Convention and/or carrying the Red Cross or Red Crescent emblem and flag, many ships were bombed, confiscated or damaged with the intent to harass. In 1917 Germany accused England of misusing hospital ships for the transportation of troops and ammunition, in essence violating number four of the Hague Convention and so declared a policy of unrestricted warfare. This meant that all ships, including marked hospital ships and other neutral vessels, would be attacked if discovered. The Germans' formidable U-boats were, therefore, given free range to destroy any hospital ship that crossed their path. In all, twenty-six hospital ships were sunk during the war, the first being HMHS *Anglia*, which struck a mine on 17 November 1915.

Chapter 1

Wounded Belgians

We stood by for the Belgians at midnight. At midnight we were told that they would arrive at 2 a.m. At 2 a.m. that arrival would be 4 a.m. At 4 that it would be 6, and at 6 that it would be 8. At 7.30 we were actually at the station, and a little before 8 we were told that the convoy would arrive at 9.

It was cold and bleak at the station, the refreshment rooms were not open, and we had had no breakfast. The hospital was about twenty minutes' walk away. Breakfast there was at 8 a.m. I decided that there would be time to walk briskly to the hospital, have breakfast and return. I suggested this to the other temporary, but he would not risk it. I did and was breakfasting when one of the regular junior MOs came in. He stared at me in surprise and asked how I came to be there. 'By Jove,' he said, much amused, 'you won't half be for it if you're not on parade.' I said that I meant to be, and swallowing my last cup of tea, started off again, arriving on the platform at 8.50. The Dug-out looked daggers at me but could do nothing since my orders were to be there to meet the train. When we arrived, we transferred the wounded to every sort of horse-drawn and petrol-driven vehicle. The townsfolk had got wind of the arrival, and a large crowd had assembled and lined the whole route to the hospital. When we loaded up the last case, one motorcar remained. The other temporary and I took this. Now at that time very few people were familiar with the sight of a British Naval officer in uniform, since officers always came ashore in mufti. As we whirled out of the station the crowd set up a tremendous cheering, which was taken up and continued throughout our drive home. Two distinguished Belgian officers no doubt! There was nothing for it but to lean back and acknowledge the compliment as gracefully as possible.

The Belgians gave us something to do – if only to censor their letters, which were in French and Flemish. One morning I wished to make a small incision in the inflamed hand of a man in my ward and asked the steward for the gas apparatus to be brought up. A steward told me in horrified tones that the gas apparatus must on no account leave the theatre. My patient, who was quite able to walk, had therefore to be wrapped in blankets, placed on a stretcher and solemnly wheeled down to the theatre.

Most of the MOs, having nothing to do, watched operations in the theatre, and there, in the presence of ten doctors, including at least one specialist, I made an incision one inch long on the back of the patient's hand, with all the pomp and ceremony of a major operation. One of my colleagues afterwards thanked me for a most interesting demonstration. Eventually, to my great satisfaction, another temporary and I got orders to join the hospital ship *St Petersburg* at Southampton. She turned out to be a small passenger vessel which normally ran between Harwich and the Hook of Holland. We arrived in the evening. The chief steward was surly and rebellious and refused to help us on board with our kit. No doubt he was missing his usual tips. Fleet Surgeon X was in medical charge of the ship and appeared to have the coldest of feet. On a fine October morning we slipped down Southampton Water, eating our breakfast on deck. We had on board some forty nurses and a detachment of RAMC proceeding for service in France.

Attached to us was a company of St Johns Ambulance men, often referred to as the St John's, a more undisciplined set of ruffians I never set eyes on. I do not mean this as a criticism of the St John Ambulance Brigade as a whole, but this section was certainly not a credit to the organisation. On arrival at Calais, they all broke ship, going ashore on shopping expeditions. When they returned the Fleet Surgeon clapped them under hatches and dismissed them on return to Southampton. We had no Red Cross sign and no escort but were probably not considered worth the expenditure of a torpedo. We had hardly berthed at Calais before Belgian wounded came streaming down the quay, some in motors and some walking, and our first concern was to get rid of the nurses, as we needed their bunks. They went off to the Hospital Sophie Battelot, but two volunteered to return with us, and very useful they were. We loaded up in the afternoon and during the night, and sailed next morning, having 577 wounded on board – a gross overload. All the bunks were full; mattresses were laid side to side in the saloon and smoke-room; patients lay in the corridors and on the boat deck. Really rough weather might have washed many overboard.

There was every class of wound from a slight scratch to fractured thighs and men shot through the chest or abdomen. These latter had to be propped up against the pillars in the saloon as best might be. The majority of the cases had been wounded several days previously and had not been touched since they were roughly tied up on the battlefield. They had lived and slept in their clothes, and the severer cases were in a deplorable state of sepsis, vermin and filth. When dressings were removed green and black fluids gushed from their wounds, the stench in some cases being almost overpowering. Our equipment for dressing wounds consisted of a torpedo-boat chest, which did not amount to much. Economy was the watchword of the Naval Medical Service. It appeared that it was the glory of the naval surgeon to return to port with his medical stores intact as on setting sail. I heard of one naval surgeon who would uses strips of an old shirt to dress a wound or make a poultice rather than expend a portion of his sacred boracic-lint. As to instruments, the Fleet Surgeon had none, nor had the other temporary. I had a pocket case and was the proud possessor of the only pair of surgical scissors on board. When in port we begged stores wherever we could, but no one was anxious to part with what they had. Having some Pot Iod and iodine crystals, we got some methylated spirit and compounded our own tincture of iodine. Once we were lucky enough to get hold of a jar of peroxide of hydrogen.

Fracture cases had been put up by entirely unskilled hands. In some cases the fragments had been fixed at right angles to their proper alignment. In others a heavy splint had been put on below the fracture, merely adding weight to the tortured limb. Fortunately, we had some chloroform and, under anaesthetic, with patients lying on the floor of the saloon, took down, straightened out, and reset the limbs, using such improvised splints as we could obtain from broken up packing-cases. By 'we' I mean the other temporary and myself. The Fleet Surgeon did nothing in the way of treatment, he divided the day and night into watches, and prowled around wondering how long it would be before we were torpedoed, but I never once saw him stretch forth his hand to help a patient.

Much of our time was spent on our hands and knees in the saloon, as to attempt to walk about without 'sea-legs' was to risk lurching heavily on to a patient. Also, we were seasick. In the course of his prowling the Fleet Surgeon came to the conclusion that there was space in the ship of which we were not aware. There were two stewardesses on board. Neither they nor the stewards did anything for us that they could possibly avoid, and for many hours of the day they were invisible. Taking advantage of a moment when both women were on deck, the Fleet Surgeon entered the ladies' lavatory and found a door leading from this into a cosy little lounge warmed by an electric heater. There was another entrance, but this had been nailed up and sealed. Here they had been living in luxury, whilst we had been cramped in the tiniest of cabins with nowhere to feed. On arrival at Southampton the Fleet Surgeon sacked the stewardesses and the stewards except two, whom he compelled to wait upon us properly in the lounge.

We lay outside Southampton for the night before berthing, which was unfortunate, as we had no rations for the wounded. The stench in the ship increased. Two patients had died before we were able to get under way at Calais, and another died before we could land him. After unloading we enjoyed the luxury of a hot bath and a couple of square meals ashore. We sailed again at 7.30 next morning, and after delaying off Sandown Bay, crept along the English coast, and about 4 p.m. lay off Dover. Having taken some 'Mothersill', I was not sick, but felt rotten, and thanked goodness that another hour should see us in port. Just then, to my disgust, I heard the anchor go down, the captain having decided that it would be dark before we could make Calais. A night on the rolling wave at anchor is no pleasure to a landsman!

We crossed in the morning, reaching Calais about 8 a.m., and there heard The *Hermes* had been torpedoed an hour previously only a few miles away. The CO from the Sophie Battelot came aboard and asked us what the devil we meant by kidnapping two of his best nurses. We pleaded not guilty, and called the nurses, who expressed their wish and intention to stay with us. The crafty fellow, however, had had their baggage removed during the argument, and they had to follow. Before leaving he promised to replace them, which he eventually did, but he might as well have kept those that he sent us.

Orders now reached us that we were only to take the more severe cases, and that the walking, or rather running, wounded were to be diverted to a ship bound for Cherbourg. They were soon swarming down upon us. As soon as they sighted the ship, those who could do so broke into a run, shouting 'Angleterre'. It was necessary to stand in front of the gangway with arms outstretched, calling out, 'Pas par ici! Par La! Bateau *Princess Clementine* a Cherbourg,' 'Angleterre,' they cried in response, 'Angleterre,' and surged upon us, so that we narrowly escaped being pushed into the dock; their one desire to place a strip of water between them and the dreaded German.

A Belgian man shot through the neck stalked aboard with much dignity, asked to be directed to his cabin, and enquired at to what hour dinner would be served. I left him to discover that his 'cabin' was a bunk, and that dinner was only a dream. We sailed again in the early afternoon with a cargo of between three and four hundred wounded. It was so rough that even some of the seafaring men were sick. As for ourselves, we were completely laid out, and at one time I almost wished that the damned boat would sink and have done with it. The state of the wounded was similar to that of those on the first trip, and much vomiting added one more flavour to the fetid atmosphere below. We lost the packet-boat off Sandown and had to put out to sea again to find it. Once more, landing was not possible until morning, and once more the unfortunate wounded went unfed.

Other voyages had little to distinguish them from the foregoing description, save that each time we returned with a smaller cargo, until at length we appeared to have mopped up every wounded Belgian around Calais. The ship was paid off, and I returned to the depot forthwith – too promptly, in fact, as I found that no one knew of our whereabouts, and I might just as well have given myself leave.

About a fortnight later I was ordered to report to the Admiralty. There I was ordered to proceed to the RNAS station at Kingsnorth, Hoo, North Kent. The station, Beluncle Halt, was not in any time-table, but the train took me there all right down the single-line. The air station was about a mile away, a desolate-looking collection of sheds on the mud flat, surrounded by barbed wire. Personnel, 150 – two officers and other ranks. Healthy young fellows, seldom sick.

Consequently, there was little medical work to do. The job would just have suited one of the old dug-outs.

Not much happened to me here, except a flight in an airship and a close-up of Winston Churchill, but I did see one of the earliest parachute descents, if not the first from an airship. The representative of the firm called to try to get a contract for the supply of parachutes. He was a nondescript little man. Asked if his parachutes were 100% efficient, he said reservedly that he had never known one to fail to open. He backed this up by offering a demonstration. No building was high enough, so he asked if an airship could go up. Permission was obtained by phone from London and a ship went up to 1,000 feet. It was blowing a great deal, but the little man jumped all right. The wind caught him, and he came down about a quarter of a mile away in a ploughed field. Shortly afterwards the representative of another firm called. Asked as to the efficiency of his goods, he said that it was utterly impossible for one of his firm's parachutes to fail, but he did not bite when a jump was suggested! Later, the commander smilingly said that however efficient this man's parachutes might be, his recommendation would go to the man who jumped.

Certain of the officers expressed a desire for anti-typhoid inoculation, so I got the necessary equipment and started on them. The air station was guarded by a company of military, and some of these I did also. Inoculation was not compulsory, and forty-eight hours' excused duty was allowed for recovery. Later, leave was allowed for this period as a bribe to the timorous.

A young lieutenant approached me, explained that he proposed to spend his forty-eight hours with the dearest girl in the world, and mentioned that he wished to appear at his brightest and best when in her company, and would I – that is to say, could it be – here he became somewhat incoherent, but it was easy to see what he was after. Leave first, inoculation afterwards! It was not difficult to wangle it. He was a decent lad, and one of those with whom I used to scrap after mess, but I made him swear his Bible oath that he would not subsequently refuse inoculation, and that he would do his best to carry on duty afterwards. He went off in great form and returned in his glee to announce his engagement. Leave must have done him good, as he took his inoculation without turning a hair.

The commander was a charming fellow, and the officers a very cheery lot, but there was nothing whatsoever for an MO to do, and nothing to see except mud, corrugated iron, and barbed wire. Had I ever been inclined to drink, I must have fallen at this time. I looked up at the little blue book that had been issued to us on enlistment and found to my horror that I was liable to serve for five years. On another page, however, I discovered that there was opportunity to resign after six months. I put my resignation in in good time, rejoiced when it was accepted and, while working my time out, obtained a post in a civil hospital.

Chapter 2

The Army

In the summer of 1915, as the war did not seem likely to come to an early conclusion, I again wrote to the War Office. This time I had a reply almost by return of post. Now when I joined the Navy in 1914, I was subjected to a most stringent physical examination, being tested minutely as to sight, smell and hearing, and made to climb a rope, hand-over-hand in a stark naked condition. When near the top of the rope, however, there came a sharp order to drop down – it appeared that the windows of a school of young ladies overlooked the examination room. In 1915, however, it was a different story. A young MO pointed a stethoscope somewhere near my chest – asked me to cough twice – said, 'You've no varicose veins, have you? No! Good! Cheerio, you're in.'

In due course I was ordered to York. There, no one told me anything, but on the following day I happened to see a list of names, which included my own, and learned that I was posted to a Lancashire Fusilier battalion at Masham. Accordingly, I discovered the location of Masham, proceeded there, and reported to the colonel in camp, stating my appointment and mentioned that I had just joined. Long afterwards I found out that the old boy thought I had said that I had just qualified, which accounted in some measure for the boorish way in which he treated me. Colonel W. might have stepped out of a picture book, even down to his small iron-grey moustache. He had been in India, of course, and the curry must have got into his liver. He was kindly at times, but he was a snob, and regarded with contempt the temporary officers who were not of his own military caste. But with all his insistence on discipline and respect, he himself was not above referring to his brigadier as 'old pudding face', even in the presence of junior officers. Later, I learned that I was the fifth MO who had been sent to him, and the first to stay the course.

I had no training whatsoever (the RAMC school at Blackpool not being then in existence) and did not know my exact position as MO. Otherwise I might not have remained with him. I first got into his black books through being truthful. He was furious. My medical equipment consisted of one stomach pump, one thermometer and boracic lint. I applied for a few simple remedies which I knew they had got at the field hospital, but all I got was one ounce of zinc ointment. I was assisted by an intelligent, but medically untrained, corporal.

We proceeded from Yorkshire to Andover via the west coast of England, presumably to teach us that the longest way round is always the correct military route. Tidworth was certainly better than Masham. The four battalions of the brigade were billeted in comfortable huts, within a few hundred yards of each other. There was room to manoeuvre and gallop about. Tactical exercises were begun in earnest. The men argued with each other as to how many times we had attacked Two Tree Hill and as to whether it had ever been captured. I soon had a row with the CO on the question as to whether I should attend to the corns of the battalion. This brought me into contact with the ADMS for the first time. He told me that I must train battalion chiropodists. I told him that I had no knowledge of chiropody. 'That doesn't matter,' he said, 'you must train them,' and with that he dismissed me.

One morning the MO of the 18th Battalion came over and asked me to go with him and help Shand, of the 23rd Manchesters, who had a large number of men to vaccinate. We went over to the Manchester lines, where there was a small hospital, and for an hour or two were busy vaccinating some hundreds of me. The hospital was within the precincts of the camp, and as I had nothing to do after sick parade and sanitary inspection was over, it did not occur to me to tell anyone where I was going. As I strolled back into our lines, I was met by a frantic orderly, who told me that I was wanted at once in the orderly room. The old man was purple. He asked me where the blazes I had been. I told him. He asked me what the devil I meant by leaving the camp without his permission. I replied that I had not been out of camp, and that in any case I was doing necessary medical work. He was in no way mollified, but continued to storm for a while, and then asked me some futile little question, for which was all he required me. Such was Colonel W., but he had his weaknesses.

We had two officers in the battalion, brothers named N----. They were gentlemen, and both had held commissions in the Navy. The elder was efficient but addicted to the bottle. The younger was similarly addicted, but less efficient. The men called them Charlie Chaplin, Nos. 1 and 2. One day a corporal, recently transferred to the battalion, had a report to make and was doubtful whom to report to. 'Go and tell the Chaplin' said a man in all innocence. The corporal stepped up to the younger Mr N. and saluting him smartly, said 'Company all present Mr Chaplin,' and was thunderstruck by the torrent of profanity that greeted that simple statement. The colonel was very fond of these two officers, and overlooked their faults many times, but eventually they both had to go. I could relate further incidents about this crusty old curmudgeon and no doubt I have forgotten many more, so it is not surprising that eventually I began a desire to get even with him.

Now on field days the MO's party had to man an imaginary aid post, usually in the middle of a field or on a hillside and hang about all day waiting for imaginary casualties – a most wearisome business, which taught us nothing. On a certain date we were notified that we were to perform night operations. To be posted on top of a windswept hill for half the night doing nothing, while the rest of the battalion kept themselves warm charging about, falling into rabbit holes and generally getting mixed up, was far from enticing. Further, we were to be done out of our evening meal – possibly to make things more realistic. I thought of it with disgust. On the morning of that day I happened to go over to the camp hospital and saw the Manchesters' medical corporal, an intelligent, dapper, little dark-haired man, Riley by name, who was a commercial traveller in civil life. I expressed my opinion of night operations to Riley.

'But why go Sir?' he said.

'Why go! You know my colonel. If we had a regimental goat he would have it out bell and all.'

'But,' said the intelligent Riley, 'a man might be taken seriously ill just before "Fall in"!'

'In that case, the CO would say, "Attend to him and fall in afterwards," and if it was a serious case, there would be little to do, save telephone for an ambulance.'

'True,' replied Riley, 'but it might be a man in my battalion.'

'In that case your MO would attend to him.'

'Ah,' he said, 'but I don't think I shall be able to find Dr Shand tonight. He's very difficult to get at in the evenings.' He looked at me with a twinkle in his eye.

'We fall in at 7.30,' I said.

'Very good, sir.'

At about 7.25 I was in the hut which I shared with young Caldwell, putting my things together. Riley had evidently forgotten. A sudden clatter outside, a hasty tap on the door, and he burst in, saluting smartly and asked if I could possibly come over to MR lines to see a man taken 'very ill'.

'Where is your own MO?' I asked, glaring at him.

'Can't be found, sir, looked everywhere. He's very bad sir, temperature 102.'

'Oh, send him a pill, Doc,' said young Caldwell.

'No,' I said, 'if he's 102, I suppose I must go and see him. Will you tell the CO if you see him?'

'Hope I don't,' said Caldwell.

I left, grumbling about MOs who could not be found. Outside Riley marched smartly for some fifty paces then slowed down and spoke.

'He's roaring with pain,' he said.

'Who?'

'Moran, down in the corner in his blankets.'

'D'you mean he is ill?'

'Just a precaution, sir, I thought someone might come in with you.'

As we entered the hospital a terrible moan came from a far corner. Riley walked over and kicked the sufferer. He sat up with a grin. But the excellent corporal had not yet completed his programme. There was a good fire in the stove, and something sizzled. Out came plates, and presently we were consuming fried potatoes and sausages. This finished, Riley opened a tin of fruit and produced a carton of cream obtained from the village. Coffee followed.

'And now, sir,' he said, preparing to clear away the plates, 'what about a little entertainment?'

But at that moment, to our dismay, we heard the outer door opening. Riley sprang across the room to defend the fort, then gave way – and Shand walked in.

'Why, what the hell!" he exclaimed on seeing me.

We enlightened him and he approved of the plot.

'What about a little game, sir?' said Riley, holding up a pack of cards.

'I don't mind,' said Shand, 'I've nothing to do.'

So, the table cleared, we settled down to a quiet game. Shand and I could have got into serious trouble for this, but as we played for no stakes, we were not doing much harm. I kept an eye on the time, however, as even Riley agreed that it would be well that I should be with the battalion on their return.

Accordingly, warm and well fed, I set out about the time that the battalion would be starting for home. After walking about two miles I was passing down a dark lane when I heard the jingle of bridles, and the CO and the adjutant rode past me as I walked in the shadow of the hedge. I let most of the column pass and fell in with the signallers under Mr Bernstingle.

'Lo, Doc. Where have you sprung from?'

As we marched home, I told him the whole tale, which amused him mightily. We dismissed on the parade ground and made for our huts. Caldwell came in done up and cursing the whole affair.

'Was the man very bad?' he asked.

I replied that I did not feel inclined to leave him and described the groans that had greeted us at the hospital.

'Poor fellow,' said Caldwell, and rolled into bed.

Next morning I was summoned to the orderly room. I stepped in smartly, closed my heels and saluted.

'Why were you not on night operations?'

'I was called to see a sick man in the Manchesters' lines, sir.'

'Why you?'

'Apparently their own MO could not be found, sir.'

'But you could have followed on afterwards!'

'I did, sir, met you, and fell in with Mr Bernstingle's party.'

'All right,' he said, glaring, 'you may go.'

Then as I went I heard him grumbling to the adjutant that doctors always defeated him, and he felt scores were about level, especially as I had beaten him the previous day at revolver shooting, an exercise at which he fancied himself. Alas, for truth, but he had taught me the art of subterfuge!

One more story concerning the old man. Every six weeks we were entitled to a weekend leave. There were four MOs within a radius of a quarter of a mile, and two of us might well have been away each weekend, but this, no doubt, was not considered good for us. Weekend leave began after parade on Saturday and lasted until midnight Sunday, or to be more correct, till 23.59 hours Sunday night. On any other day of the week I could have got away after breakfast – sick parade being at 7 a.m., but on Saturday mornings I had a louse parade at 11 and, however smart you may be at your job, it takes considerable time to inspect the hands, bodies and feet of 1,000 men.

Once I managed, by arrangement with the company commanders, to do the louse parade on Friday afternoon, but the old man tumbled to it, and on the next occasion put on another parade at that time. Now it chanced that I had the opportunity of a lift into Salisbury, where I could catch a good train. The only snag was that I would have to leave camp before the CO had signed the leave roll unless he signed it early. He did not. It was most desirable to get away early, as it was a good three miles to Tidworth station, and the only means of transport being Shank's pony. Trains were infrequent, and the journey to London long and slow. I waited until the last moment, and then decided to chance it. I walked on to the platform at Salisbury, and there was the Colonel! There was nothing for it but to take the bull by the horns, so I went up to him, saluted, and bade him good evening. He was in high good humour.

'Hullo, Doctor, where are you off to?' he said.

'On leave, sir,' I said boldly.

'Splendid! So am I. Make the most of it.'

Whether he had signed the leave roll or not I did not know – nor cared – for at that moment the train came in.

While at Tidworth a young officer named H. joined us. He had been to France and had been slightly wounded in the arm. He was a well-educated, somewhat slightly built, loose-limbed youth of nineteen, but he stood six feet in height. The Colonel appointed him assistant adjutant, gave him leave twice as often as anyone else, had him sit next to him at table, and generally made a fuss of him. As might be expected, the youth had got a certain amount of swelled head. One morning we were to go out about 4 a.m. for some field exercise. It happened that I had a rather nice chestnut mare as my mount. Before leaving H. said to me, 'I'm going to ride your horse today Doctor.' I made no reply but thought that he might at least have gone through the formality of asking me to lend him the mount, even though he may have considered his position in the unit entitled him to have it.

Having gone no great distance we entered one of those broad grassy lanes that are common in that part of England. On one side was a bank and hedge, at the foot of which was a shallow muddy ditch, through which ran a sluggish stream of water. Rank grass grew out of the ditch, that nearest the bank being about eighteen inches high. There had been heavy dew and the grass was wringing wet. On the opposite side was a belt of fir trees, with a way through them leading to a large open space of ground. The main body passed through the opening and disappeared. I remained in the lane along with a section of men and one or two more details. These men were standing at ease in two ranks with their backs to the fir trees. I was on the other side of the lane with my back to the ditch. I did not need my horse, so told the groom that he could take Jess home instead of hanging about. This would also conveniently avoid any argument as to who was to ride her. Presently, H. came striding through the gap, looked expectantly round, and scowled.

'Where's your horse, Doctor?' he asked.

'I sent her home, I did not need her.'

'But I wanted to ride her,' he said, stepping over to my right.

'Perhaps you did,' I replied dryly.

'Damn you,' he exclaimed, and with that he seized me by the neck with both hands, his right on the throat and his left at the back of my neck, which he could easily do, as he stood head and shoulders above me.

I said, 'I will give you two seconds to let go, H.'

He grinned and increased the pressure. I counted two, and then let into him. To anyone from the North of England, it was perfectly simple to turn sharply to the right, grasp him around the lower part of the chest, swing in a cross buttock, and at the same time fling him from me. His hands left my neck and shot up above his head, and he flew through the air like the famous young man on the trapeze, straight for the ditch. His right hand ploughed up the liquid mud, which was shovelled up his sleeve and plastered all over one side of his body. In addition to this the sopping grass drenched him. He picked himself up and made as through to rush me. I fell into an easy crouch. But after advancing a couple of steps he swung round and strode off through the opening in the tree. It was only then that I realised the presence of the section of men. They were doing their best to stand properly at ease, but it was taking them all their time. The Colonel's groom had buried his face into the horse's neck, his shoulders shaking convulsively. I had thrown the adjutant (and the Colonel's pet) into a ditch in the presence of the men! The words 'contrary to the maintenance of good order and discipline' came to mind. But it couldn't be helped! The whole cavalcade shortly appeared through the trees, and we went back to camp.

After foot inspection I retired to my hut to await the expected summons to the orderly room. It never came. Either young H. had sportingly attributed his dirty condition to an accidental fall, or else he must have quietly told the Colonel the truth, and the old man may have been amused and have chaffingly advised him to let doctors alone. At all events I never had any more cheek from young H.

Returning to quarters one night, I was surprised to find a strange individual in Caldwell's bed, and a quantity of kit strewn over the small space in the hut. The stranger introduced himself to me as a major who had been transferred to us. I remarked that Caldwell would hardly be amused at the arrangement when he returned from leave. 'Then he will have to make the best of it,' said the major. Sometime after midnight Caldwell came in, stared at his bed and blinked frowningly round the hut. We exchanged greetings. 'And who' said Caldwell stepping forward, and speaking with rising indignation, 'who have I the honour of entertaining in my bed?'

'Major Sir Henry --- -----, Bart, MP!' barked the individual, sitting up suddenly.

'Good evening, sir,' said young Caldwell, and proceeded to make himself as comfortable as possible on the floor. I admired his restraint. Had it been myself I should certainly have been on the mat the next day.

Sir Henry stayed with us for several days, which made things very cramped, since he had a full-size batman and any amount of kit. He was very affable and invited us to help ourselves to his excellent cigarettes, which we did, and so also I fear did our batmen Hodgins and Crook. These two men were marked 'Home Service', much to their disgust. Before we went out, the ADMS vetted the home service men and passed a number for general service. The list was given to me for fair copy and transference to the orderly room, typed copy to be returned to the ADMS for signature. I summoned Hodgins and Crook and asked them if they really wanted to go to France. They stoutly affirmed that they wished for nothing better. It was simple to insert their names, but a disability had to be stated against each. Crook was three-parts deaf. This could be minimised, but Hodgins' difficulty was vision – he had never been able to put a shot on target, and great importance was attached to musketry. Later, it was so neglected that a man would throw a bomb at impossible range rather than attempt to use his rifle. I told Hodgins that he must have flat feet, which he replied, 'Very good, sir. Both feet, sir? Yes, sir.' He was a prodigious liar and a wonderful thief. You only had to think of something you might want and Hodgins would go out and steal it. Our hut was better furnished than any in the block, and that was how the major came to be billeted upon us. All went well, and shortly the two men were going about swelling their chests and proclaiming themselves to be foreign service men. Hodgins made further ineffectual attempts on the target, and the sergeant major tore his hair. I say all went well, but at that psychological moment Hodgins lost his job, and continued thereafter to lose one job after another.

In France, in losing a job he invariably paraded before me in full marching order, grounded arms, and asked what he was to do next! Apparently, from his point of view, I was solely responsible for all operations on the Western Front. The old devil knew perfectly well that I had got him to France under false pretences.

He was, successively, batman, stretcher-bearer, padre's orderly, cook, storeman and watchman. When I made him a watchman I felt that my stock of jobs was running low, so I told him he must hold this position, as otherwise, I should be obliged to shoot him. 'Very good, sir,' said Hodgins, and fortunately he did retain this job as long as I was with the battalion.

France loomed nearer, and Sir Henry's batman requested a private interview. He was Sir Henry's valet in private life and was drawing both civilian and military pay. Asked what he wanted, he said that he did not think his sight was too good and mentioned something about a little business that his brother-in-law was getting together. I told him that if he wished medical attention he must report sick at the usual hour. He made the regulation reply, and then had the audacity to murmur about it being worth £5 to me! I advised him to leave my quarters before I made up my mind to report him to his master. He reported sick next morning, and I gave him a chit to the hospital, where they supplied him with glasses which he never wore. He was rightly served in the end, for when Sir Henry was wounded on the Somme he was not allowed to return to England with his master, but to soldier on.

Chapter 3

France

Early in the winter we were served out with pith helmets and believed we were bound for Egypt. The helmets were withdrawn, however, and we subsequently went to France, landing at le Havre early one morning. I had two men sick and dumped them with the landing staff. Once disembarked, we were marched right across le Havre and not by the shortest route apparently. Though it was mid-winter the day was blazing hot, and the men were wearing their greatcoats, besides being encumbered with all their equipment. They cannot have slept much and had had little or no food since the previous afternoon, so it was not surprising that they began to show signs of exhaustion. We encouraged the little men (they were bantams) to put up a good show before the French, but the accursed paved roads seemed to be endless. At one halt a man, having taken of his equipment, seemed quite unable to resume at 'fall in'. In a rash moment I seized the equipment and threw it over my shoulder, though I had quite enough of my own to carry. It was a grave error, as at the next halt the man could not be found. I did, however, get rid of the bundle eventually.

At last, we arrived at camp where everyone began to settle down, when to the general disgust, the whistle blew for 'Fall in'. We were in the wrong camp and had to retrace our steps across le Havre. Some optimist in the battalion called out, 'Are we downhearted?' to which the sturdier spirits in the company replied with the usual lusty negative. One of the men in blue shouted back, 'then you soon ---- well will be.' This is an old gag I know, but it was literally true in this case as, on rounding the next corner, there arose before us what must have been the longest and steepest hill in all Northern France.

The camp was on the hilltop, a most exposed spot. I won't attempt to describe the ascent of that hill, but it was an appalling struggle. The band had their instruments with them, and halfway up the big drummer fell in some sort of a fit. He had been cursing the --- drum and saying that it was just ---- murder and wishing that he could just be shot right away. Accommodation = bell tents. The CO took the officers into town for a meal and delighted himself by displaying his few words of French. The night was as bitterly cold as the day had been warm. Young Caldwell and I lay back to back on the bare tent boards in an effort to keep warm. A gale of wind and a stampede of horses added to the night's entertainment.

Next day the men entrained for St Omer, and were eventually billeted in a small village, the name of which I have forgotten. In a day or two I had two sick men who required hospital treatment. We were not in touch with the Ambulance Corps and had received no instructions as to the disposal of the sick.

I found out that there was a military hospital in the town of Aire, a few miles away, so we hitched up the Maltese cart, laid the sick men in the bottom, and the medical corporal nipped up beside the driver. I got hold of a map, mounted my horse and trotted in front to guide them. We found the hospital and left the sick men there, fortunately not coming into contact with anyone in authority. Afterwards, I got a wigging for doing this, but when you are without orders and things are urgent, you have to do the best you can. Our medical equipment was very limited. Iodine was our chief standby.

One morning a lad came with tonsillitis. Not having any efficient gargle, I took a long-haired camel brush and painted the back of his throat with tinct: Iodi. Some of the men outside saw this and said, 'Blimey, he's shoving it down their ****** throats now!' The patient, however, came back for further application, so it must have done him good. The men said that they would all be doctors after the war, as it was evident that all you wanted for a 'doctor's shop' was a box of No. 9s and a bottle of iodine. They called me everything from a 'B-----dy old sailor' to the 'Iodine King'.

We were provided with two large oblong boxes, or perhaps they should be called baskets, iron-bound, covered with a sort of fabric, and very heavy. They were modelled on the South African War and contained very little that was of any use to us. The most modern article in them was dated 1905. At first, I used to drag these medical panniers into the line with us, but I soon learned wisdom and we carried all that we really used in dressing-bags and haversacks. At a later date a benign shell relieved us of both panniers, much to our joy, as it lightened the cart and made more room for kit. The useful stuff was, of course, in our bags. The panniers were forgotten until one day a personage from the back areas came to inspect us.

'Where are your medical panniers?' he asked.

'Destroyed by shell fire, sir.'

'What! No panniers!' he cried. 'You must indent for some at once.'

We thanked him but said that we did not wish for any – in fact, would rather be without.

'Nonsense,' he said fussily, 'you must have medical panniers. I will see that you get some.'

And get the accursed things we did and had to drag them about with us for the rest of the war. Don't let us condemn them altogether – they were useful to sit on!

The old man made me Mess President – without the option, and gave me 100 francs to start with, telling me to send out bills to the officers at regular intervals. (Of course, that most invaluable person the Mess Sergeant had been left at home in England.) I sent out the bills alright, but none ever paid them, for the very good reason that no one had any money, the field cashier arrangement not yet having materialised in the division. The CO drank a large quantity of whiskey at intervals (he did not get drunk) and smoked heavily, and he expected his piton and cigarettes to come out of the mess fund. One hundred francs went nowhere, and I soon exhausted all my own money. When I applied to him for more funds he swore and asked why I had not sent out the bills. I said that I had done so and informed him of the negative result. He was very keen on preserving the regimental mess. He must have been thinking of Brussels and the eve of Waterloo, as battalion mess was impracticable at the front. The majority of the officers favoured each company having its own mess.

On the next occasion on which I applied to him for money to carry on, he swore again and asked what I had done with the last lot. Thoroughly fed up, I replied:

'If you and the adjutant drank less whiskey the money would go farther.'

He denied that he drank the bulk of the whiskey and said that all benefited equally in the arrangement that whiskey came out of the mess funds. It was pointed out to him that quite half of the officers did not touch it. He then said that they ought to – and might have made it an order if he dared. This was about the last straw and the company messes were formed.

I did not get rid of the HQ mess president job, however. One morning, as we were about to set sail for a field day, the CO came up, said that he wished to entertain the inspecting general to lunch, and told me that I must get something to eat. The only thing that we could get at short notice (or perhaps our money could buy) was a string of sausages. The day was wet, and those sausages were 'cooked' – that is to say, just nicely warmed, over an open fire. Hungry men, however, are not too critical.

I was violently ill that evening and spent good part of the night with my head over a bucket, but even in that miserable state I wondered whether the general was also regretting our CO's hospitality! Next day we moved – myself on an empty stomach – and on arrival at our destination, still loathing the thought of food, I decided, rebelliously, that the old man could get his own supper as far as I was concerned. I had found my billet when I met Layman, a subaltern who had been a medical student. He told me that he had found a cosy little pub and induced me to meet him there after dark. Accordingly, about 8 p.m., we were in the best room of the little establishment, and to our joy found that stout was sold there. More than that, the landlord produced some very nicely-cooked steak. Now my all-day fast had gone a long way towards a cure and the desire for food had begun to return. We spent a very comfortable evening. Next day the CO asked me if I was still sick last night. I said that I had not completely recovered. He grunted something, but glory be! I got the sack as mess president.

While at this place we were inspected by Lord Kitchener. The inspection was to have taken place just outside the village, but this was altered at the last moment to another spot some miles away and we moved off in the pouring rain down roads ankle deep in liquid mud. Eventually, we were formed up on a muddy field at the roadside and stood there sinking in the ooze. Lord Kitchener was more than an hour late, and when he did come he hardly left the road. Afterwards he and the CO took up a position to the left of us and the battalion moved to the left in fours to march past, wheeling to the left again as they passed him. It was a most ill-chosen position, as an open ditch ran across just short of the saluting base, and the unfortunate little men had to give eyes right and stride across the ditch at the same time. Quite a number of them fell down in the attempt. Colonel W. was aggrieved that Lord Kitchener did not take more notice of him and expressed the opinion that his Lordship had deteriorated greatly.

Chapter 4

Richbourg

We went into the trenches for the first time at Givenchy, for instruction with the Royal Welsh Fusiliers, a band playing 'Keep the Home Fires Burning,' as we left la Gorge. It snowed heavily, and our rations did not arrive. The Royal Welsh, however, generously shared their rations with our men who repaid this kindness by (accidentally) shooting one of the R.W. sergeants through the stomach!

Our NCOs were chiefly old regular reservists and at Givenchy one of these took unto himself the bulk of the platoon's rum ration. He was found crawling on his hands and knees in the snow along the bottom of the trench. The old man, who, as I have said, really had a heart, was loathe to court martial him, as he feared that the sergeant might lose the service pension he had already earned. He managed to arrange matters so that the sergeant was reduced to the ranks without the pension being interfered with, and the next parade presented the odd spectacle of a man over six feet in a line of men, none of whom stood much above five feet, and commanded by a sergeant of the same dimensions! We went into the line on our own at Richbourg l'Avoue. The CO made most of the watermen into bombers and sent my sanitary corporal away on escort duty. It was necessary to invoke the aid of the ADMS to get my personnel restored.

In trench warfare the Regimental Aid Post was a fixed position usually in the support line, and the incoming and outgoing MOs handed over to each other independently of the battalion relief. Regimental stretcher-bearers (drawn from the men of the battalion) elected cases and brought them to the RAP. A squad of RAMC bearers was attached to each RAP and the RMO handed his cases over to these men, who carried them to the advanced field ambulance or to the next relay post if the distance to the AFA was too great. At the AFA they were seen again by an MO, who transferred them to the field ambulance by horse or motor ambulance. From the field ambulance, cases went by motor convoy to the casualty clearing station, several miles farther back, usually out of range, where operations were performed. At about the same distance as the CCS were Corps rest stations, where medical and skin cases were treated. After assortment at the CCS cases were taken to the railhead and so by hospital train to the base.

At Richbourg the RAP was in a fairly well preserved house, about 300 yards from the front line. The back of the farm was towards the trenches, and the front of the house looked on to a road running parallel to the front line. About 300 yards to our left, along the road, was a much dilapidated farm, which housed BHQ. Down the road to the right stood a ruined factory, and from Factory Corner, another road called the Rue de Bois, ran roughly at right-angles to the line. Usually the cases were brought down the Rue de Bois, but it was not a good route, as the line curved to the right of us, and brought the road under crossfire. Sitting in the farm at night we would hear a machine gun begin to mutter, and then as the gun swung round, the noise of the spray of the bullets striking the end wall of the house. Also there must have been a fixed rifle somewhere, with a patient individual sitting by it, as from darkness onward, a single bullet would strike the wall with monotonous regularity at intervals of about one minute. The road between us and BHQ was traversed by rifle fire, and the old man said that the only thing that amused him about the place was that the doctor got shot at every time he came to the mess. Incidentally, I had to pass the grave of another doctor on each of these expeditions.

Having become familiar with the sector, I prospected for a better way of getting wounded from the line and found a route under cover practically all the way, entering the aid post from the rear. The only snag was that behind the farm was a fairly wide ditch. We got some timber and made a bridge, and for a time all went well until the brigade ammunition carriers discovered our bridge, used the route, and further, made a dump of bombs at the RAP. Hitherto, we had been left in comparative peace, but two mornings later, we were shelled to blazes. After two direct hits, which hurled bricks all over the yard, I thought it time to make a move and, collecting the men to make a dash for it, sent Corporal Holmes to the RAMC shelter, to warn them that we were about to abandon the post.

It was needless. The RAMC had already fled, one of them running all the way to St Vaasy, some two miles away! We waited for the next burst and then sprinted for the BHQ. I reported the matter to the CO, who took necessary action, with the result that the dump was removed and we were shelled no more, which seemed to indicate that the Germans knew that the place was the aid post and were willing to let it alone, as it was not used for any offensive purpose.

At one side of the yard was an archway filled up with sandbags. One morning an MO from the field ambulance came up and, looking round, told us to remove the sandbags and use the archway as an entrance. I mentioned the machine gun which played along the wall. He did not seem to think that it mattered – it wouldn't to him, as he would never be there at night – and said that we should have an opening there, as we might be trapped in the yard (which was absurd). I said that I would bear his remarks in mind, and as soon as he was gone gave orders that no one was to touch the sandbags. He must have come up again, however, as on our next tour in the sector, we found the archway opened up, but it was significant that the outgoing party had only removed the sandbags on the last afternoon of the occupation. Opposite the archway was an outhouse which was used as a latrine. I gave an order that no one was to use the latrine that night and sure enough, next morning the wall all across the doorway was splattered with fresh bullet marks about head high. We built a buttress outside the building, in line with the archway, but no stretcher-bearer brought a case in that way – they knew better!

At this place, Private Tinning, one of my orderlies, was seized suddenly with diarrhoea and vomiting. In spite of treatment he did not improve much, and developed a peculiar grey colour. Then all his teeth began to get loose. In our antiquated equipment we had some perchloride of mercury tablets, which we dissolved to make an antiseptic lotion. I asked him had he been using any of the surgical vessels for drinking purposes. He denied this but later said:

'Oh Sir, you know that there blue ointment? I've rubbed myself with that.'

This was unguentum hydrarg, which was used for a very local purpose. Now Tinning had become lousy for the first time in his life, and was too ashamed to report it. He had seen the ointment used for local pediculi, and concluding that it would be lethal to the body louse also, he lathered his body plentifully with the 'blue butter', so poisoning himself by inunction. A good bath removed the source of the poison, but the mercury had got well into his system, and by the time that he was again a fit man, we were all lousy!

While at Richbourg, the battalion did a raid. The CO was worried and very anxious that everything should be done to make the affair a success. Two days before the date it appeared that there would be snow. The CO decided that the men must wear white overalls and sent a mounted officer into Merville to get some. All the officer was able to procure were some two dozen French night-dresses, complete with frills. When the men learned that they would be expected to wear these things, their language was quite unprintable! It did not snow and the dresses were never used – that is, unless the old man himself wore them!

We had a nervous little padre attached to us, and this individual expressed a desire to be in the front line at the time of the raid. The CO at first flatly refused, then he weakened and said that the padre might go, placing him in my charge. Padres can be very useful, but they can also be a great nuisance. Of course, this one was missing when we were ready to move off, and I was faced with the choice of abandoning the line or being absent from the post of duty at zero hour. We were just going without him when he rushed up.

Halfway up the communication trench we stopped to rest. The trench was near the Rue du Bois and subject to crossfire. As we sat there I saw a head and shoulders raised above the level of the parapet. At such moments one speaks to soldiers in language that they understand! 'Keep your ---- head down you --- fool!' I barked. The head disappeared; there was a low chuckle at my side. 'That was Parson, sir,' said Corporal Holmes.

The raid had little result save casualties. The CO was here, there and everywhere, trying to do everyone's job, and wanting to know exactly how much blood had been spilled, when he would have been much better in a central position receiving reports. His out-of-date ideas were exemplified one day at Fromelles. A party of men were ordered to leave the road and take cover in some trenches about 50 yards away. They set off at the double. 'Don't run men,' said the old man, standing in the middle of the road, still convinced that the British soldier should remain upright, until shot down by the enemy. If he had seen what I had seen, a few days previously at the same spot, he could scarcely have objected to the men running. He was personally brave enough.

One day, tired of struggling along a trench, he said to his orderly, 'Come on Smith, we've only got to die once, we may as well go over the open.' 'All right for 'im,' as Smith said, ''E's an old man, but I'm only twenty-five, I am, and I 'ope to 'ave a bit of fun yet.' The exposure told on him, he became more irascible, and even the adjutant (an ex-regular colour sergeant) turned upon him and said that he would not be spoken to like a dog. At Fromelles in April he left us. He had done his bit in the war, and had had the satisfaction of taking his battalion into the field.

Chapter 5

Neuve Chapelle

Our new CO, a regular soldier, was a spry, alert looking, red-haired man. I called him The Fox. Leaving Fromelles, we arrived one evening in a small village behind the lines. HQ mess was in a farmhouse, the aid post being in the barn across the yard. Over the barn was a loft in which the HQ orderlies were billeted. We had hardly settled down when there was an urgent call from the aid post. I went over and found a certain Corporal Sharples with blood spurting from his eyeball in the same way water spouts from a burst pipe. We fixed him up and sent him off.

There happened to be a company of grave-diggers in the area, and one of these men, an Irishman, had been in the habit of sleeping in the loft. On this evening he had retired to the loft in an intoxicated condition, to sleep there, as usual but soldiers can be extraordinarily unkind to each other on occasions. The HQ men resented the presence of the stranger, and Corporal Sharples twice flung him to the floor. After the second assault the Irishman picked himself up and swung wildly with his right, connecting with the corporal's head. The first interphalangeal joint of his right index finger (i.e. the first joint beyond the knuckle – the fist being closed) must have fitted itself to the outer angle of the orbit, and have swept across the eye, crushing the eyeball against the inner wall of the orbital socket and bursting it. The colonel's servant, who was a boxer, then stepped in and knocked the Irishman out. The HQ orderlies made out that the Irishman had been the aggressor, but I got the true facts from my servant Crook. I told Crook that he ought to give evidence as to what he had seen, and at the trial noted that he formed one of the prisoner's escorts. He was not called, probably much to his relief. The unfortunate Irishman, who cannot have remembered much of the events of the evening, got twelve months, and the corporal got home to England at the expense of the loss of an eye.

Soon after that we went into line at Neuve Chapelle. Here we were pestered by rats, which had plenty to feed on, as many bodies had been built into the parapets or buried in shallow graves. If they did not actually run over you at night, they would fight amongst the sandbags and send cascades of earth over your face as you tried to get off to sleep.

Our rest area was Vielle Chapelle, a few miles back but not out of range. One fine evening a sing-song was held in the yard of the Brasseries, where the men chanted their usual dismal ballads, about blind mothers, lame sisters and dying parrots! I don't know whether this attracted attention, but next morning a shell fell on the road between the Brasseries gate and the canal side. A French civilian and a serving maid were killed and a British gunner wounded. I picked up the gunner, and bound him up with a silk handkerchief, which was all that I had. In addition to these, poor Madame la Brasseries had most of her hind quarters shot away, and died in the field ambulance an hour or so later.

My billet was a small estaminet owned by a carpenter. When we first arrived, the landlady and her daughter burst into a torrent of speech, out of which I translated the words, 'She was not ill, only very old, not ill at all,' and gathered that the grandmother had recently died in that bed that I was to occupy. I told them that dead grandmothers held no terrors for me, and all was well. The carpenter was very friendly, and when all was closed up for the night, he would regale us with his secret store of wine. He was far too polite to make any charge for this, but his courtesy also prevented him from refusing the money which we offered. He shook his head over the casualties. 'Four coffins in one week! It was terrible,' he said, but no doubt privately thought that is was good business.

When in rest at Vielle Chapelle, we supplied working parties for the line at night. On an evening when one of those parties was up the line, an orderly came behind my chair at mess and whispered that Lieutenant X. would like to see me. On enquiry as to where he was to be found, I was surprised to learn that he was in his billet, as I knew X. to be the officer in charge of the working party. I found X. lying face downward on his bed, his head in his hands. He told me an incoherent story of how, when he had got his men to the appointed place, the enemy had 'put down a curtain of fire,' and said that his men had been killed right and left. After this he had become confused and finally an artillery officer had told him to return to Vielle Chapelle. The poor chap had come to the end of his tether. He had not been fit when we were in England and, for some time past, I knew that he had been struggling to keep a grip on himself. I had the unpleasant duty of reporting the matter to the adjutant and then to the CO. The Fox was bloodthirsty. His ginger hair seemed to stand up straighter than ever. He was all for putting X. under immediate arrest, and I believe would have liked to shoot him there and then. I stuck it out that it was not a case for arrest, maintaining that X. was not mentally responsible for his actions. After some argument, the CO ordered me to call Colonel Dick, of the field ambulance, for consultation. This colonel's real surname was Richard, but everyone called him Dick. Colonel Dick viewed, and agreed to take the officer into hospital. The CO took the decision well enough, and wrote a detailed report to the brigadier, mentioning Colonel Dick's name several times. Only when the report had gone did he realise what he had done, and was obliged to send a wire to Brigade begging that, in recent correspondence re Lieutenant X., the brigadier would in all cases for 'Dick' read Richard. X. was sent down the line, and the battalion saw him no more, but sometime later a paragraph appeared in the paper stating that he had been dismissed from the service, the King having no further use for his service as an officer. I often wondered if the poor wretch was eventually conscripted as a private soldier. At all events, he escaped the firing party.

Chapter 6

Dentistry

At Vielle Chapelle I had the pleasure of drawing a tooth for one of the few really pretty girls that I ever saw in France. To do this it was necessary for me to conduct her personally through the village to the aid post, as a sentry stood on the old drawbridge over the canal with orders to let no civilian pass. Corporal Holmes was very enthusiastic over the operation, and tried to induce her to return for further treatment!

One most useful thing we had in our equipment was a folding leather case containing five pairs of dental forceps. I used to put the case in my pocket when going round the line, and many a tooth did I draw in the front trench, the patient sitting on the fire-step with his back against the parapet, and myself with a knee on the step for steadiness. No anaesthetic of course! It was wonderful how the men stuck these bald-headed extractions, sometimes having two or three out at a sitting, and then returning for more!

While at the same place someone suggested rugby football, though it was hardly rugby weather, and word reached me at the aid post that a party had gone down to see what they could do. Anxious not to miss a game, I followed, and found some officers and men on a piece of flat ground. Heaps of stones and clothing served as goalposts and the crossbar had to be dispensed with, but at least they had a ball. They were just ready to kick off, so I pulled off my tunic and leggings and joined in the fun. Getting a pass on the left wing I went off down the touchline, failing to notice that the said touchline was one of those shallow stagnant ditches that separate the fields in France. Going 'all out,' I was well tackled and pitched headlong into the green slime, to the great entertainment of all ranks. This put me out of the game, and I returned to the village.

News travels fast. I found Crooke sitting grimly on the step on the estaminet! 'Your bath's ready, sir,' he said, looking at me more in sorrow than in anger, but at the same time managing to convey that none but the most devoted batman would remain with such a lunatic. I spent the rest of the afternoon cleansing myself in the 6-foot canvas bath, which took up most of the small space in the deceased grandmère's bedroom, while Crook waited to soak my clothing in the bath water.

At Richbourg once more. An NCO reported sick. He arrived with full equipment, in evident anticipation that he would be sent to hospital. Asked what he complained of, he said that he was 'Done, finished, could soldier no more'. He showed no signs of exhaustion or even of fear, and examination failed to reveal anything the matter with him. I ordered him to return to duty. He left the room, but later finding that he was still in the building I spoke to him severely and told him to be off. He went, but again returned. Asked why he had not obeyed orders, he said that he was unable to return to his company. 'Very well,' I said, 'I am going up towards your company to look for a well. You can come with me.' I took him up the Rue de Bois to the point where the communication trench branched off and watched him go up the trench. Continuing up the Rue de Bois, I found the well and returned to the aid post.

I had not been gone long, when my friend was back before me. I wasted no more words on him, but reported the matter to the CO at lunchtime. The Fox acted promptly and the man went back to duty under escort. In the afternoon the CO went round the line and spoke straight to the man, telling him that it was better to chance a German bullet than to make sure of an English one. We had no more trouble with this man. He had had his 'try on,' and it had failed. Weeks later, on the Somme, I came upon him sitting calmly in a heavily shelled trench. He was eventually killed by a fragment of shell which passed across his throat. The Fox was much upset by this incident, and said that it was all due to the fact that Lieutenant X. had not been shot, but the cause lay much farther back than that.

When in the Fromelles sector, there was in the battalion a regular CSM for whom the old man had a soft spot. During some shelling this man suddenly turned tail and fled headlong down the communication trench, through the support line and out of the trenches altogether. Not content with this, he jumped on a lorry passing through Sailly-sur-le-Leys, and got as far away as possible from the fighting area. We never saw him again, but it was known that he had got a job at the base, and the men said:

'Now we know how to get clear of this here trench warfare. Join the regulars, get made CSM, and beat it when the shelling starts!'

The case of my obdurate friend the NCO reminds me of an incident concerning Dr Young, of the 18th Battalion. A man reported sick in line without apparent cause. Young ordered him back to duty. The man said that he could not and would not – go.

'You know what will happen to you if you don't,' said Young. 'You'll be shot.'

'I'd rather be shot,' said the man. 'Now?' said Young, looking at him grimly. 'Yes, I'd rather be shot now than go back.' 'Right! Up against the wall! Ginger, get me a rifle.' Ginger, half-witted and wholly devoted to Young, jumped to it, but the man had taken to his heels and was back in the front line in record time.

We were leaving Fouquiers for a town some miles away, and an ambulance was to call to pick up our sick and follow the battalion. I had a sick man with a temperature of 102 who appeared to be a TB case, so as the ambulance had not turned up at the time of departure, I left him in the charge of the corporal to await its arrival. It did not arrive, and the sick man struggled along after the battalion, arriving in the town about dead beat. The military hospital refused to admit him, as he had not been through the usual channels, and made him trail to the field ambulance on the outskirts of town, there to have his name put in a book and be sent back into town again. Red tape for ever!

We were sent to Béthune to be fattened up for some Somme slaughter and were billeted in the École des Jeunes Filles. The band played in the courtyard every morning at 10 a.m. Sick parade was at 9, and many men came up for such dental treatment as I could give – organised dental service not yet being in operation. At the suggestion of the corporal, I put back the dental cases at the end of the parade, and then at the proper signal attempted to emulate Sequah by extracting teeth to music.

At this place I had a remarkable personal escape. Some of us were amusing ourselves in a house and I was standing on a chair with a tumbler of very thick glass in my hand. Tyhurst, a wild Canadian was waltzing about the floor. Suddenly he shouted, 'Goal for Ireland,' and aimed a high kick at my hand. The toe of the boot caught the base of the glass, and the rim being driven against the lower surface of my chin, the heavy tumbler was smashed to atoms, except for a useful bruise, I was unhurt. But next time Tye shouted, 'Goal for Ireland,' I dived under the table!

Chapter 7

The Somme

Sometime in July we departed for the Somme, arriving at Avuley Wood without rations, so that we were glad to eat a few broken biscuits that we found in an old tin. We lay there for three days awaiting our turn to go in at Contalmaison, but were then reprieved and eventually went into action opposite Guillemont. Before going into the line we lay for a day or two in a narrow valley named Talus Boise, called by the men Death's Valley – and not without good reason. The valley was pitted with large shell holes, but no shells fell there at this time. We moved up to the Montauban-Maricourt road and went forward from there into the trenches, my battalion being in the front line and Shand's in support. Shand and I had a common aid post. This was a track running at right angles to the front line. On our left was a bank of earth about three feet high, on our right a high breastwork, and at this point the breastwork formed a bay, the floor of which was the roof of a German dug-out some fifteen feet below. The stair was too narrow to take wounded down, so we worked on the top. There was no overhead cover. Here we worked for three days and nights, dealing with an almost continuous stream of wounded from the attack on Guillemont. At time shells passed over us from three different directions, and Shand remarked that it would only be a matter of time before one dropped fairly into place.

During the first day, when shelling was brisk (as it nearly always was), our attention was attracted to a man coming up from the left rear with something in his hand. He was rushing forward and flung himself flat to escape the shell bursts. It was obvious that he was making for our post, and with a final dash he rolled himself panting over the lower bank. After inquiring my name, he handed me an envelope marked 'Urgent'. Withdrawing the paper, I read: 'Please inform me as early as possible – your age last birthday,' and there followed a string of questions almost equally absurd under the circumstances. I looked from the document to the messenger waiting for me to initial the envelope, and saw that he was regarding me with some apprehension. Probably my feelings were reflected in my expression! I told him to rest in a comparatively safe corner and gave him a definite order not to attempt to return until things were reasonably quiet.

Later in the day The Fox was wounded, but not too badly, and Sir Henry took over command. In the evening things became more lively still, and at one time I was in the embarrassing position of having an unwounded British officer sprawling on the ground at my feet, clinging to my knees, and imploring me for God's sake to stop the noise. I sent him off out of the way as early as possible.

Later, Norcross, one of my bearers, arrived in a somewhat similar condition. Norcross was a bad hat, and likely to try anything. I put him on one side to rest, but as he continued to kick and squeal, I went over to him and told him that if he was not quiet at once, I would send him back to the trench immediately. He was quiet at once – good evidence that he still had himself under control. So quiet was he that I forgot all about him until I walked over him in the dark, when he sat up with a genuine scream. He returned to duty the next morning.

Sometime next day a rumour reached me that a number of our men were lying wounded in some part of the line and not getting attention, so, picking up a dressing-bag, I set off for the trench but had not gone far when there were footsteps behind me. It was Tinning. 'Never alone, sir,' said the good fellow. 'Not while Tinning's alive.' We reached the trench safely, where we found Sir Henry sitting out in front of his dug-out, apparently thoroughly enjoying the war, to which, however he referred in uncomplimentary terms. He knew nothing of the supposed casualties. Soon there was a shout of 'Stretcher-bearers,' and we hurried off. Turning a corner, we came upon a wounded man lying in the bottom of the trench, which at this place was cut in the chalk and had no parapet. We were in the act of bending over him when a shell burst on the very edge of the trench, sending us sprawling over the casualty, but not harming us. Having fixed up all the casualties of the moment we made our way back to the aid post. As we came in sight round a corner, Holmes' dirty face expanded into a broad grin of welcome, and Shand, coming forward, asked me where I was hit. I told him I was not hit. He then told me that

I had been reported dead. Someone had seen the shell fall apparently directly upon us and had concluded that we were na-poo. I reflected afterwards that no one had troubled to go and look for us.

In the afternoon Sir Henry was wounded in the leg, and abused me soundly for cutting up his expensive field-boot to get at the wound. Captain Crook took command. On the third night my battalion was withdrawn, and Shand's lot took over the front line. We left about 9.30, and an hour or so later the expected happened. During a lull, Shand lay down on the top of the German dug-out. His three orderlies were lying on the track, which was on a slightly lower level, and two shellshocked men were sitting on the low bank. The shell must have landed directly on top of Shand. He was blown through the roof of the dug-out down into the space below. The spread of the explosion passed over the three orderlies, but killed the two shellshocked men on the bank. Shand's arm and thigh were fractured and one of his feet was blown off. They must have had a terrible job getting him out of the hole. He died in the early morning at Corbie.

We retired to Talus Boise, where I got down to it underneath the Maltese cart. Thirty or forty yards away a large fire was burning, on top of which rested an iron dixie filled with water for tea making. Round the fire was a group of men from one of the companies, chatting with comrades who had been left out of the line, it being at that time the practice not to take the whole strength in. The fire may have attracted the attention of a German gunner, who may have loosed off a venture, or perhaps it was just a bad shot, but the shell fell right into the fire, hurling away the dixie, scattering the embers in all directions and plunging everything into darkness. Screams and cries filled the air. I scrambled out from under the cart and promptly fell into a bramble bush. Next I tripped over some barbed wire. Then, having found my torch, I made towards the sounds. The first man I came upon had both thighs broken, and was so frantic with pain it was difficult to deal with him. This was not made any easier by the Padre, who kept tugging at my coat to attract my attention to another case. That shell killed six and wounded ten, the big drummer, who had been left out of the line, being cut right in two.

A couple of nights later we again went up to the Mountauban road to lie in reserve. Our guns were all over the place on both sides of the road. A lot of American ammunition was being used at this time, and much of it was defective, many shells bursting prematurely, some almost at the gun mouth. We had just stepped off the road into a trench when there was a loud explosion, followed by a cry of 'stretcher-bearer'. We scrambled over the top and saw in the dusk two figures, one standing, and the other crouching against his legs. The upright man had his arm practically blown off, and the kneeling one was doing the only possible practical thing, gripping his comrade's upper arm to control the brachial artery. A tourniquet was put on, and luckily an ambulance passed down the road at that moment. The explosion killed two other men. Curious to know the position of the gun that had fired, I returned to the spot in daylight, and turning around, found myself looking into the muzzle of a gun! Curiosity satisfied!

Chapter 8

A Month's Rest

Withdrawn from the line, we set off at 4 a.m. for Montaigne-sur-Somme, where we were to have a month's rest, the band playing as we marched through a small town, a sanitary man deputising on the big drum. We expected to entrain after a short march, but the train never materialised and the men who were more heavily laden than they should have been had to march all day in the boiling sun, with practically no food, the cookers having gone by a different route. The battalion, less those who had fallen by the wayside, arrived in the village at 8 p.m.

The month's rest was but a dream, and within a week we were again on our way to the line. As I sat on my horse a puffing-billy approached the head of the column. The horse pricked his ears and shuddered. Then, as the traction-engine came nearer, he curvetted, so that he stood across the road, tail to the drop. He commenced to back, slackening the reins, I slid my legs back and touched him with both spurs. Instead of moving forward he sprang suddenly backwards. His hind feet went over the edge and up went his head. Luckily, I retained my balance, leaning forward till his ears nearly touched my face. The slightest jerk on the reins would have brought him over backwards. For a moment he was poised almost vertically in the air, and then he fell sideways to the right, landing in the field and rolling on me. I grabbed the bridle, but he was too quick for me, got his head up, and started to rise. Out came his offside foreleg, the hoof plunging into the turf a few inches from my nose. Covering my face with my left arm and lying still, I did not see what happened as he rose, but was told that he lashed out with his hind feet, his hooves skimming my body. It is popularly supposed that at moments like the above, a précis of one's past life passes through the mind. My only thoughts in mid-air were: 1) 'I shall break my right leg,' and 2) 'The CCS is only two miles away.'

Tyhurst was roaring with laughter. 'Good God, Doctor,' he shouted, 'I thought you had broken your blinking neck. What do you mean by falling out without orders?' The horse was got back into the road at a convenient place, and scrambling up myself, I remounted, little the worse for the adventure.

We had arrived at the Montauban-Marcourt road once more. It was dusk. Farther down the road the AFA had a large dug-out or sunken shelter, roofed with tree trunks and heavily sandbagged. I walked down the road to call on them, to find out if there were any new arrangements for the evacuation of the wounded. It seemed that I had gone too far, so I retraced my steps. Still I did not find the place, and was looking about me in the failing light when I found that I was standing on the edge of it. The shell of the place gaped before me. The roof had been torn off, and in the cavity arms and legs protruded from a mass of rafters, sandbags and broken stretcher poles. Two shells had fallen simultaneously, one on the dug-out and one in the trench alongside. Eight orderlies, two MOs and all the wounded had been killed.

We lay in the trenches alongside the road for some days waiting to go forward. The sun blazed down and the dead in the wrecked dug-out began to make their presence known. Bluebottles settled alternately on the corpses and on our food. I asked the CO if I might have a score of men to cover the place, and so give them a temporary burial. The CO looked across at the spot, discovered that it was a yard or two outside the battalion area, and refused to allow anything to be done. Red tape had triumphed once more!

My post was at the top of a long rise, and from this point the ground sloped very gradually forward to Angle Wood, in front of which the battalion lay. A serpentine trench crossed the space to Angle Wood. This place was littered with bodies of the French, some crouching on hands and knees still grasping their rifles, others in grotesque attitudes. When passing a body near the edge of the trench, swarms of flies and bluebottles would rise from the corpse.

Returning from an expedition to the battalion position, I was complimented by having half a dozen shells fired at me personally. The trench which ran at right angles to the line of fire was only about hip-deep at this point, and I did some fine hurdling along it over fallen stakes, dead Germans, and other debris, a huge cake of earth catching me between the shoulders and helping me along. Here a man was wounded in a ghastly manner. A shell explosion blew him on to a heap of ammunition, and the ammunition then exploded. All four limbs were broken, he was hit all over the body, and wherever he was not wounded he was burnt. He was perfectly conscious, and his cries were unnerving. It was impossible to give him proper treatment, since in his frenzy he tore off the bandages as we tried to apply them. I gave him a full dose of morphia, but without effect. His cries and struggles were having a bad effect on some lads who were passing forward, and realising that he could not possibly survive such wounds, I filled the syringe again, and in a few minutes he was at peace. We buried him in a shell hole.

I now began to have a lot of pain in the back but put this down to having slept on a heap of stones. Late on the next afternoon one of my bearers was carried in, shot through the face and mouth. His tongue had swollen, so that he could neither speak nor swallow, and he desperately wanted a drink. He patiently wrote suggestions on scraps of paper, but all to no purpose, and he had to face the two-mile journey to the AFA with his thirst unrelieved. As they lifted him he shook hands with me in a curiously final manner, and for the one and only time at the Front, I had difficulty in not bursting into tears. I knew that I must be definitely ill, and sure enough a few hours later I had a pretty useful rigor. It rained as we withdrew, and slipping about on the mud, I was pretty short of breath. At the road, I crept into an empty dug-out, and in the morning, having a splitting headache, dosed myself with aspirin and quinine before we moved right out of the battle area. After marching three miles the horses met us. Mine was standing by the edge of a pit some fourteen-feet square and about the same depth. I asked the groom to move him farther away.

'Oh, he's quiet today, sir,' said the groom.

'Never mind,' I said, 'I have no ambition to roll about in the bottom of that pit with him.'

The horse behaved well enough, and we reached Happy Valley without incident. The groom took the horse and led him aside to mount him, but hardly had he touched the saddle when the animal threw him neatly over its head. On the Sunday I went out for a ride with Tyhurst, and returning about 5 p.m. held a sick parade. During the parade I was seized with most violent abdominal pains. I finished the parade and left the tent, but had not gone far when my legs became undisciplined, and I staggered about like a hopelessly drunk man. Twice I was nearly down, then the sun began to go out, and the ground got up and hit me, just as Crook and another ran to my aid.

Afterwards the CO said that I had spoiled a perfectly good Church parade by my antics. I hung on for another couple of days and then Young, of the 18th, came down, had a look at me, and sent me down the line. Young and one other were now the only two remaining of the MOs who had come out with the division. Hodgkins helped me into the horse ambulance. 'Best of luck, sir,' he said, 'an' don't be in too much 'urry to come art 'ere agen. 'Ave a week or two in Angleterre.'

Chapter 9

The Dreaded Fever

The Trench Fever, for such it proved to be, from which I was suffering, landed me somewhat unexpectedly in England. This trouble, of course, due to the louse. This little beast, carecring over the body of the man, and biting him, causes him to scratch, and so doing rubs the filth of the insect into the abrasions, thus inoculating himself with the virus of the disease. What is it like? Well, take a bad dose of influenza and double it, and you have trench fever. A feature of convalescence is the incidence of terrifying dreams, which are persistent, and far outstrip reality in their fearsomeness.

The horse ambulance took me to the field ambulance in Corbie, (France) where, to my amusement, I found myself at first treated with suspicion, and them placed on a stretcher, and sent to the CCS by motor. This ambulance drove at a breakneck speed (or so it seemed) over the bumpy French roads. I was the only occupant, and was more than once flung clear of the stretcher. I thanked heaven that I had not got a broken limb, and wondered if the driver bore a grudge against me for being the sole cause of his journey. The hospital train took us to Rouen by night. Everything in that train was piping hot. How I longed for a cool drink! A cup of lukewarm tea would have been a godsend. But I had reason to be thankful, as I peeped over the side of my top bunk, and saw poor mangled fellows lying in the bunks below. On arrival at Rouen, in the early hours of the morning, we were rushed up to the hospital, where we were literally flung into bed. I do not think that the staff of that particular ward was expecting a convoy, for presently, the regular army sister (known by her scarlet cape) came strutting down the ward looking anything but amiable. Pausing near my bed, she said crossly, 'What's the matter with you?'

'I understand that I have been marked PUO,' I replied.

I did not tell her that I was an MO, as I did not want any preferential treatment, nor did I disclose the fact to her at any time during my stay there. No doubt she was wilder than ever when she discovered it for herself.

This alphabetical nomenclature was a constant source of speculative interest to the men. PUO (Pyrexia of Unknown Origin) was thought to mean 'Patient under Observation'. ICT (Inflammation of Connective Tissue) they translated 'I can't tell' – a candid confession of the ignorance of the medical services (Military Branch), while NYD (Not Yet Diagnosed) became 'not yet dead,' but NYDN mystified them completely.

I never realised before how much I loathed boiled milk, and that was my staple diet. One morning as the MO made his round, I asked him if I could have a cup of tea.

'Certainly,' he said. 'You know it won't do you any harm.'

'I do,' I replied, 'but here I am under orders.'

In any case I would never have asked that woman for anything. I got my cup of tea, but not from her, and 4 p.m. became the golden hour of the day. It was only one cup and a biscuit but it was grand. Some mornings later the MO asked me, 'How are you?' I always felt better in the mornings and naturally said so. (It was in the evenings that the complaint gave you a gee up.) On this morning after I had replied, the sister suddenly burst forth, 'He always says he is better, but he is not well yet,' at which I realised that she must be human after all!

At the end of the week, I was up, and to my surprise someone told me that I was marked for the hospital ship. I had lost my hat on the journey down the line, and before leaving the hospital one of the nurses crammed a hairy purple affair like a large tea cosy on my head. As I boarded the ship I heard someone remark that he now believed the rumour about the Russians having passed through England!

On arrival at Southampton we were asked where we lived. Thinking it hopeless to mention my home in a remote part of the north of England, I mentioned a town in the Midlands. They promptly sent me to the Isle of Wight.

At the Isle of Wight we were fed and housed sumptuously in the Old Queen's house. Having eaten a good breakfast, I set out to 'tramp across the island,' but found that my walking powers only took me to the far side of the lawn, where I sat gasping on a bank. After a period of sick leave, I was sent to Sunderland marked 'Light Duty'. My orders were to report to Major Q – a regular RAMC officer, and not knowing under what conditions I should find him, I dressed myself as a mounted officer should. As soon as I saluted him, he told me off for wearing spurs, admitting at the same time that I was correctly dressed. I retorted somewhat tartly that I found it the easiest method of carrying them. Had I not been wearing spurs, he probably would have told me off from a different angle. He then continued, 'You have been sent up here for Light Duty – let me tell you there is no such thing.'

Life in Sunderland was not bad. For a time, I assisted the SMO in his office, and afterwards was sent out on relief work. Not far from the office there was a VAD hospital, in charge of which was a very excellent surgeon, Morrison by name. He was a very small man, quick, and alert, and possessed the tiniest of hands together with the maximum of manual dexterity. I was sent over to this place once or twice to give anaesthetics, and found such favour with Morrison that I was subsequently asked for by name. It was a pleasant change after the rough work in France, and it was a pleasure and an education to observe his technique and skill.

One of my relief jobs was at Whitburn, where a second-line artillery unit was stationed, commanded by a courtly old colonel, who, whilst maintaining discipline, made life as pleasant as possible for all under his command. At my first sick parade, fourteen men turned up complaining of diarrhoea. I gave them all a mixture of opium and castor oil, a filthy concoction to take, but excellent therapeutic treatment. Only one man returned next day for further treatment. He got something more palatable and a period of light duty. After a few days the adjutant spoke to me one day in the mess, commenting on the satisfactory fall in the sick rate:

'Do you know,' he said, 'I think there must be something wrong with our MO. Last time he was on leave the same thing happened.'

And so it was, as I discovered. The MO was an elderly man, and very sympathetic. The men called him 'No duty, John', his favourite prescription for men reporting sick being two days' no duty. Men having an unpleasant parade in prospect would wait until twenty-four hours or so before zero hour, and then remark, 'I'm not standing for this. I'll go to Old No Duty. And get clear of it.' The infection even spread to the officers, who would stand outside their huts in their pyjamas on a bleak morning, in order to raise a slight temperature.

Before my time was up, about 100 men were brought to me for examination as to their fitness to return to the front. The majority of the men had been very slightly wounded, and some had been home as long as eighteen months, their wounds having long since healed. I passed about 80% of them fit for general service. A week or two later I was in a hotel at Roker and, in the course of conversation, an officer, to whom I had been introduced, asked me, over a drink, where I was stationed. I said I had been at Whitburn. His face lit up suddenly, 'By Jove,' he said, 'are you the fellow who passed those men GS the other day?'

'Yes,' I said, 'I did examine some men.'

'Have another with me,' he cried, extending his hand. 'I've been trying to get some of those blighters back to France for months and months.'

There was another side to the picture, however. Several times at different places I prevented obviously unfit men, who had been out once or even twice, from being sent back to the Front. They were not popular with the stay-at-homes, and were often willing enough to go. The stay-at-homes were not at all to blame for being where they were. The staff of camps would not allow valuable men to leave if they could help it.

Still in the Roker district, I was looking after a battalion at Stansfield Schools, when one afternoon I was called to see a man who was throwing fits. The poor lad had been wounded in the head and had a large saucer-shaped depression in the region of the right temple, scabbed over in the centre of the depression. The area was denuded of bone, and the pulsation of the brain could be seen through the scar.

He had been turned out of a London hospital and sent back to his unit, the hospital authorities having told me that they could do no more for him. Manifestly unfit for any further service, he now lay on the floor of the bare schoolroom throwing one fit after another, a misery in himself, and a horror to the other men who were upset by his struggles, and the drumming of his heels on the floor. It was easy enough to get a man into the army at that time, but mighty difficult to get anyone out. Only a travelling medical board could do it, and they must see the man. They did not come round too often, and if I sent this man into hospital, he would miss the Board.

As it happened a TMB was due at HQ next day. During one of the lad's lucid intervals, I asked him to endure one more night in the schools, explaining to him, and to the men, that I would then be able to help him more effectually. I took him before the Board on a stretcher and they quickly marked him 'E' which meant immediate discharge. Then, having got him out of the military clutches, I had him carried round to Hammerton House, and placed under Dr Albert Morrison's care. Morrison was a remarkable surgeon and at once took the greatest interest in the case, and proceeded to perform a series of remarkable operations.

The first thing he did was to dissect the adherent skin away from the brain tissue. This stopped the fits. A portion of the dura matter – the silky covering of the brain – had been torn away (by the wound). To repair this Morrison took a piece of the fascia lata, or muscle sheath of the thigh, which he successfully grafted to the torn edges of the dura. When this was healed, he tackled the gap in the bone. Turning back the pericranium (the silky covering from which the bone regenerates), he trimmed the edges of the bone, and bevelled them so that the inner table projected slightly beyond the outer. Covering the wound he then went to the other extremity of the patient, and removed a thin portion of bone from his shin, together with an overlap of periosteum. Bevelling the edges in the opposite way to those of the skull, he fitted the piece in position and sutured periosteum to pericranium.

This operation lasted three hours, during the whole of which I kept the patient under chloroform and ether. The graft took well, and in time the boy had a sound bony covering. He had no more fits. One more operation remained – a skin graft to cover the wound, but the series had taken many weeks, and before this could be done I had returned to France. This was not the only case of the kind cured by this surgeon. I saw one lad twelve months after his cranial repair. He was quite fit and well.

Eventually I handed the schools over to another MO and returned to HQ. The SMO ordered me to go around all the hospitals in the town and discharge any men who were fit for duty. This work was mostly done in the afternoons, and I must admit that I timed my visits so that the inspection would finish about the tea hour. They make good tea in hospitals, and the sugar ration was no problem for them. Taking one hospital a day, I had cleaned them up by the end of the week and reported to the SMO that the job was done. He seemed rather annoyed. Regular MOs are terrible dawdlers and he probably expected me to take three times as long over it. He told me shortly to go and live at a certain hotel, and be on call. I asked for forty-eight hours' leave, but he refused, saying that he wished me to be on the telephone. I went to the hotel and the next week of my military service was spent chiefly in the picture houses of the town.

I was then sent to a place called Cotton Hall. The officers were accommodated in a country house with all modern conveniences, a comfortable room, a bathroom handy, a well-appointed lounge, excellent fare and very little work. It was 'Home from Home,' but much too good to last. After a week or two I was summoned to HQ. The SMO told me that he wished me to exchange units with a Captain Claymore, who was at the Hilton Castle. He explained that Claymore had suffered from dysentery, and had had two operations on his lower bowel, which had rendered him incontinent. The latrines at Hilton Castle were at some distance from quarters, and were of the usual draughty army kind. Anxiety about having to turn out in the bitter night was aggravating Claymore's incontinent condition. I, of course, agreed, and the change was made. I only mention this because it has a bearing on subsequent events.

One day called to a sick man, I had a sudden hunch that the moment I saw him that he was suffering from spotted fever – the dreaded scourge of camps and prisons. Examination of the patient supported this opinion, though he had, of course, no spots at this stage. I sent for the ambulance, and while waiting for it, rounded up the man's platoon, had him isolated in one hut, and took all precautions. When the ambulance came, I gave the driver a chit to the SMO with notes on the case an ending 'CSF?' At the same time I told him that he was on no account to remove the patient from the ambulance until he had been seen by Major Q. Half an hour later I was called to the phone. Major Q. was at the other end in a great state of excitement. Yes, he thought it was cerebro-spinal – was practically certain and he proceeded to give me a string of orders. I was, however, able to assure him that I had already tied all the knots in the 'Red Tape.' I don't know what became of the patient, but am glad to say that we had no more cases in the camp.

There were always a certain number of men in these camps who were quite unfit for further service. Travelling medical boards would descend on us like bolts from the blue. AFB 179 had to be made out for each case. These forms had to be obtained, and the men could not always be produced at short notice. After one particularly hectic scramble to get ready for the board, I sent in a request that I might be provided with a few AFB 179s, so that I could vet the men at leisure, and have all written up in readiness for the next board. I was curtly informed that on no account could I be permitted to have any of these forms and that any in my possession must be surrendered forthwith. Not long afterwards, I had equally curt orders to indent at once for a supply of the said forms, with a veiled suggestion that I had been neglectful of duty in not applying for them sooner. You must not think for yourself in the army. You must let authority think first, or at least you must let authority *think* that they have thought first!

Chapter 10

France and the Third Battle of Arras

Late one forenoon the SMO rang me up, saying, 'You're to go to France tonight.' I started to pack, and was just snatching a bite of lunch when the major himself appeared to say, 'not tonight, but this afternoon.'

'What about embarkation leave, sir?' I asked.

'Out of the question,' he said, 'I've brought an ambulance to take you and your kit to the station.'

So that was that! Arriving in London late, I found to my disgust that under the DORA regulations I could get no food, and that the hotels were full. Determined to have a decent night I waited until the people were turning out and then slipped into an empty lounge, turned out the light, and got down to it on a big chesterfield. In the morning, after a wash and brush up in the lavatory, I walked into the breakfast-room with all the assurance of a resident. Breakfast was all that I paid for.

I went out with several other MOs. One, a man of fifty, was furious at being sent on foreign service. Another groaned that he was nigh on sixty years of age. The old boys were terrified that they would lose their luggage and could not be persuaded that the ROD would see to it that they and their luggage arrived OK. The hospital at Camiers was our destination. Here, one of my first jobs was to receive convoys of wounded and sort them out. In the early days of the war, every sort of case that was fit to travel (and many that were not) was bundled off to England. A little later, with better hospital organisation abroad, the lighter cases were kept in France. Later still, when hospital accommodation abroad had been extended, with more complete equipment, the pendulum swung back again, and light cases went home, while a large number of severe cases were kept for long periods in France.

On the threat of an offensive in the area served by any particular hospital, the majority of the cases could be quickly evacuated. In 1917 the classification of cases with which I had to deal was, Hospital Ship A, B, C, or D. and convalescent camp. HSA was helpless cases. HSD was deck cases. Con. Camp cases remained in France. The distinction between HSD and CC was a fine one. In order to be methodical and to achieve a degree of equity, I asked all borderline cases how long they had been in France, and the date of their last leave. Any man who had been out twelve months or more or who had not had leave for many months, I marked HSD. I believe that the great majority of these men answered me truthfully – indeed they did not have much time to digest the purport of the questions, but the CO soon sent for me, and said that he wished to inform me that it did not follow that because a man had been wounded, he must be sent to England.

Early one morning my ward took in part of a convoy. Going round, I found a lad who had had a good part of the back of both thighs shot away. He had to lie permanently face downwards. The damaged tissue had been cut away at the CCS, and the cavities filled with gauze salt packs. Long strands of cat-gut passed from edge to edge of the wound, over the pack, keeping it in position. I started very carefully to remove the gauze from the right limb, but even with greatest gentleness, it was a painful process. I had nearly finished when an Australian staff nurse came up, and without being asked, started on the other leg. Grabbing the scissors at her waist, she lashed through the catgut and roughly tore the long roll of gauze from the wound. The poor fellow screamed in agony, 'Doctor! Doctor! Oh! Oh!' he cried.

'Ah ha!' said the nurse grimly, 'it's not the doctor that's got you now!'

God preserve the wounded from such Ministering Angels!

I was soon sent up the line, a fact which incensed my fifty-year-old friend, who wished to protest against 'this injustice'. The poor chap had not yet realised that he was in the army. The order – to find the ADMS 56th Division – was so urgent that one might have imagined someone bleeding to death at the other end.

At Étaples, the RTO said take the 7.30 and get out at Bouguemaison – good advice, for the train went no farther – but not a word would he breathe as to the whereabouts of the division. From there, I lorry-jumped, inquiring as I went, and after fourteen hours of travelling, finally ran the ADMS to earth in Arras, at about 8 p.m. He was expecting no one. I had beaten the military post by two days. He fed me and sent me on to the

FA, where at 10 p.m. I stretched out on a bare floor, and was soon fast asleep.

The field ambulance was located in the Hospital St Jean, in the town. Though damaged, the greater part of the building had survived. I was in time for the third battle of Arras. The out patients' hall was used for reception. A double set of rails was placed parallel to the right-hand wall. Incoming stretcher cases were placed in rows across the rails. One end of the room was curtained off, and here there were trestles, on to which the stretchers were lifted in turn for attention. After attention, the stretchers were lifted, and again placed in rows, across rails down the left-hand side of the rooms, to await removal to the CCS Entrances, right and left, made this arrangement work smoothly.

On the day of the battle, up to 1 p.m., we had a steady flow of cases. After that the rate slackened suddenly. The reason was that our first troops had succeeded, and then had been driven back, leaving the helpless wounded behind. A fresh advance recovered many of the cases during the next few days, and for a fortnight cases from the initial attack continued to dribble in. Many of the helpless wounded were cases of fractured femur, and it was interesting to observe their physical condition on arrival, with reference to the time factor, and the amount of exposure which they had undergone.

Classification might be made as follows:

GSW FRACTURED FEMUR

Cases	Condition
Picked up early Splints applied	Good
Picked up early No Splint	Poor
Found after forty-eight hours Splint applied	Good
Found after forty-eight hours No splint	Very Fair
Found after many days *Few* cases had splints!	Fair

This may seem somewhat strange, but it is capable of perfectly reasonable explanation. A fractured femur is associated with a great amount of shock, and the mortality of cases from the cause (i.e., from shock) was appalling. The man removed at once without a splint, was still suffering from the initial shock of the wound, and to this was added the secondary shock of very painful transport. The man removed at once with a splint still suffered from initial shock, but had comparatively little added shock. The man, who had lain out for forty-eight hours, had had time to get over the initial shock, before the ordeal of transport.

The month was May and the weather was fairly warm. The effects of exposure were not marked. Even men brought in a week after wounding were in wonderfully good condition. Fortunately, for the wounded, it rained soon after the attack, and they were able to collect rain water in their ground sheets for drinking purposes. For food, they ate their iron rations, and those of the dead near them. I saw one man who had lain out for thirteen days. He was very weak, but not done for. The poor fellow had been forced by thirst to drink his own urine.

The Hospital St Jean had been an important hospital in peace time, and as the operating theatre was intact, someone suggested the somewhat novel idea of performing major operations on urgent cases at the FA. For this purpose, a surgeon and three nurses (volunteers) were imported from the CCS. The selected cases were abdominal wounds, where the time factor was important. It was useless, however, as the unfortunate men on emerging from the anaesthetic and finding themselves still under shellfire, suffered from such a degree of added shock and disillusionment as to more than counteract any advantage that might have been gained from early operation. The matter was settled when one morning a shell went through the nurses' bedroom. No one was there at the time, but it was enough. They were full of pluck, and wished to remain, but the CO wisely ordered them back to the CCS.

Whilst there, I heard a strange tale about an MO. He had never been in a forward area, and was ordered to Arras. In a day or two, his corporal reported that the MO was not well. He was found with pin-point pupils, and outer signs of morphia poisoning. On revival, he admitted having taken a large dose of morphia – saying that he had no intention of serving in a forward area (or as he called it, in the front line). Placed under arrest, he was put in a small room with an orderly constantly sitting beside him. All articles were taken from him. He asked if he could have his watch. This was given back to him. Later, the orderly, glancing at the patient, was startled by the extreme pallor of his face. Getting no answer to a question, he pulled back the bed clothes. The bed was a pool of blood and near the patient's hand laid the watch-glass broken in half. The MO had felt for the pulsation of the femoral artery, and had deliberately and steadily scratched through the tissues with the sharp edge of the glass until he had opened the huge vessel; a more determined case of suicide would be hard to imagine.

One night, as we sat at mess, a series of large explosions commenced. As they got louder and more frequent, we thought that the Bosche was giving us an extra ration of shells. A huge dump of ammunition a few streets away had caught fire and it was going up in cart-loads. Several of us ran upstairs and watched the show from the upper window. The sky was lit up by the huge bonfire, variegated every few seconds by clouds of purple, yellow and green smoke. Crash after crash thundered out, varying in intensity with the number of shells that went off at one moment. The dump contained small-arms ammunition, rockets, and Very lights, as well as heavy stuff, and the crack of rifle ammunition was added to the din, while there was such a display of fireworks as I never hope to see again. Discretion being the better part of valour, we soon left the window; indeed, we were needed elsewhere.

The burning shells were hurled all over town by the explosives, and soon a dreadful procession began to arrive in the hall. Men carried, men limping, and men dragging themselves into sanctuary, and lying on the floor or sitting up against the wall, patiently waiting their turn for attention. Seeing one rather elderly man crumpled in the corner, I went over to him. 'It's all right, Doctor,' he said, 'I'm not too bad. I can wait a bit.' This, though he had some half-dozen wounds.

The dump caught fire about 8 pm., and the explosions continued until midnight. It was calculated that more ammunition went up that night than was used in the whole of 1915.

Chapter 11

Myself a Hospital Case

After a turn in the forward-bearer post, which was dark, damp and lousy, being in caves some fifteen feet below ground, we went back to the place called Warlus. Here, I was 'lent' to the Corps Rest Station, which was full of ICTs and PUOs. ICT was a kind of impetigo, which was most prevalent between the knee and ankle, due, I believe, to the wearing of puttees, and other coverings of this part of the anatomy. The ordinary soldier had the following layers of clothing below the knee: long under-pants reaching to the heel, a thick stocking pulled up to the knee, khaki trousers folded round the leg, and several yards of puttee wound tightly over the lot. The local perspiration must have been great and lice must have found a comfortable billet in this area.

HQ was in a shady wood with white ducks parading under trees. We were bombed one night and, as orderly officer, I got up to attend to things. *Some* bombs they must have been, as though they were quite a distance away, they seemed to be right on top of us. Coming through the wood, I felt myself burning all over, and wondered if I was getting the wind up. Next day, before lunch, I crawled into my hut and my afternoon temperature rose to nearly 104. I dozed, but at the same time, by a great effort, I could always open my eyes. At the same time I dreamed. One moment I would be a Red Cap controlling traffic and would push any heavy lorry which disobeyed my signal into the ditch with one hand. A great effort and then I would see the green trees and the ducks and think what an idiot I am. Then eyelids would droop again, and I would be taking fly-kicks at machine guns, which were annoying our troops. Another effort, and once more the trees and the ducks.

The CO sent me over to the château and from there I went, by stages, to the base at le Treport. At each stage the procedure was the same – castor oil, and other medicines, which made you sweat. Down came the temperature, the nurse smiled and said, 'Now you're all right!' and forty-eight hours later, up went the temperature again. This went on for seventeen days. I was not very happy at the base, and when a few days after I was out of bed, the major sent for me, and asked me how I was, I said 'Fit'.

'What do you mean?' he asked.

'Recovered,' I said, 'I wish to return to my unit.'

Now this was no Spartan heroism on my part, but because my current year of service was nearly up, and I would shortly be due for 'contract leave,' which I knew I should never get so long as I was in hospital. Warning me that 'my blood be on my own head', he marked me 'duty', and I proceeded to dig shrapnel out of German prisoners, who endured the process with utmost stoicism.

While there, I met a noted gynaecologist whom I had known in Edinburgh. He was delighted to see me, and at once asked me to give anaesthetics. 'Not much in your line here,' I remarked. 'No,' he said, 'but I'm lucky to be doing surgery of any sort, and just now I am very glad to see an Edinburgh man. All the fellows here are afraid to give chloroform.'

Up the line once more! At Étaples I saw a familiar-looking figure descend from a train. It was Claymore. Our destination was the same, so I suggested that we take our time, telling him of my journey to Arras. Travelling by easy stages, we took a week getting to the line, and even then were not expected. The FA, to which we were sent at Rosenthal, had no room for us, and we were told that we could sleep on the floor of the mess. The mess room was one storey up and, the door being nailed up, entrance was affected by a window, a short rickety ladder being placed under this. Waking in the morning, I asked Claymore what sort of a night he had had.

'Pretty fair,' he answered, 'but I had to go down into the garden for the usual purpose.'

We moved that morning, marching through Dunkirk to St Pol. St Pol consists mainly of a long pavé street. On the left, or land side of this, were plenty of houses; on the right fewer houses and beyond them a long expanse of sand. Between these houses, sandy lanes ran off the main street. Claymore and I were billeted in a tall red house on the right of the road, to get to which we had to pass through a door in the garden wall. Our two narrow rooms each had a French window overlooking the sandy lane.

We were a jolly party at mess that night, and all had a few drinks afterwards. Someone asked Claymore how he liked the ambulance. He replied with a remark intended to be complimentary. The Acting OC, an Irishman, took the remark in the wrong sense and for a moment it appeared that they might come to blows. Peace was preserved, however, explanations followed, and shortly afterwards we left for our billet. Halfway up to the house, Claymore stopped and said, 'Do you know, I don't think that fellow understands? I had better go back and see that everything is all right.'

'Very well,' I said, and went on to bed.

Later, I heard Claymore come heavily upstairs and go into his room. About 2 a.m. I woke suddenly. Moonlight was streaming into the room, and all was quiet. I was wondering why I had wakened when a voice, which seemed to come from the bowels of the earth, called out 'Orderly'. 'Claymore,' I thought. 'I'll let him in,' then realised that I had already heard him come to bed. 'Dreaming,' I thought, and settled myself for slumber. But again came that sepulchral voice, 'Orderly! Orderly!' No doubt this time! I went to Claymore's room. The bedclothes were turned back, and the window open. Looking out, I saw Claymore, in his pyjamas, lying out on the sand twenty feet below. Slipping on boots and a tunic, I went to him, and asked what happened. 'Don't know,' he said thickly. 'Pain in my backside. The old wound. I'm done for this time. Help me in', or words to that effect, for he was very 'inaudible.' (drunk)

With great difficulty I got him into a sitting position, and then on to his feet, propped against a wall. He was a heavily-built man, weighing sixteen stone. I then got him across my back, grasping his wrist over my shoulder, and staggered with him to the door in the wall. Inside the garden he groaned out 'put me down, for God's sake,' and slid down by the wall of the house. I went upstairs for a pillow, and then went over to the mess for help. Snores greeted me. The OC and second in command were lying comatose, with a bucket between them. No help there! Stretcher-bearers? At a farm about half a mile away! Clad as I was, I went, and beat upon the first tent with a stick. An angry head appeared. By luck it was our own orderly. 'Turn out a squad,' I ordered, 'an officer has had an accident.' On reaching the lane, I said, 'Through here,' and pushed open the door in the wall. We entered the garden.

There was no one there! I was staring blankly at the spot where Claymore had been, the bearers staring somewhat resentfully at me, wondering, no doubt, whether the new MO had shell-shock, when suddenly in a patch of moonlight, two figures appeared clad only in their shirts.

'Who are you?' I challenged.

'Northamptons, sir,' (I was in temporary charge of their battalion encamped on the sandy plain, and no doubt the two had crept out of their tent, for a more comfortable billet in an outhouse.)

'Have you seen anything of an officer?'

'Yes, sir, we carried him inside.'

Going in, I found Claymore, well covered up, lying on a mattress, placed obliquely across the floor of the small kitchen. He declined to be moved, but complained vaguely about one arm, which was somewhat swollen. Dismissing the men, I went to my room, only to find that all that remained of my bed was the iron work! The remedy was obvious – I got into Claymore's bed.

In the morning I was wakened by a loud altercation in French and English, followed by shouts, thuds and groans, from the stairway. The French couple, in descending, had narrowly missed stepping on Claymore's face. 'They could not have "a malade" lying across their kitchen – he had some dreaded disease without doubt.' The orderly and Monsieur had then seized Claymore and were now heaving him up the stairs. We got him into bed. He was very helpless and in much pain. At breakfast I reported the trouble to the OC. He and the second in command came across, but were unable to throw any light on the events of the night.

'What do you make of it?' asked Claymore when they had gone.

'This,' I said, 'you wanted to make water: went to the window for the purpose and being sleepy (tipsy) tipped out over the sill.'

'Nonsense,' he said, 'I should have broken my neck.'

'You ought to have done, but you did not.'

'Rot.'

'Remember, I heard you come to bed, and then found you lying on the sand.'

'No, no,' he said, 'this is what must have happened. I would feel the call to go down to the garden. I must have slipped on the stairs, catching my buttocks on a step. That would also account for my arm.'

'Very well,' I retorted, 'if you went to the latrine in the garden, why did you afterwards open the door in the wall, walk out into the lane, and lie down.'

He shook his head.

At night he was very restless. Every half-hour he knocked on the wall for me. I would go in, change his position, give him a drink, and light a cigarette for him. Shortly before breakfast, as I lifted him into a more comfortable position, he looked up gratefully, and said with some astonishment:

'How the hell can you lift me? I weigh sixteen stone.'

My own fighting weight at that time was about nine stone, seven pounds. During the day as I sat with him, he said suddenly:

'Do you know, I believe you are right! Do you remember the place where we spent the night at Rosenthal? We entered that room by a window, of the same type as this one, but not so high up – with a ladder underneath. Waking up, I must have seen the window – thought it was the same one – and stepped over the sill expecting to find the ladder.'

I nodded. He had fallen on sand certainly, but below the window there was a doorway, and projecting in front of this a flat slab of slate, serving as a step. He may have hit this. He was sent to the hospital, but before he went he gave me a sum of money for the two men who had helped him. I notified the AP corporal that I had something for these men, but no one ever reported to claim it. Claymore, however, wrote to me from hospital that he had missed his watch, and the loose cash that had been in his clothing. From England he wrote, enclosing a sketch of his pelvis, as shown by X-ray. It was fractured in two places, and one of the carpal bones of the wrist was dislocated. Exit Claymore.

My year was now nearly up, and I was asked to sign a fresh contract. I replied by applying for the leave to which I was entitled. Sign the contract, and you shall have leave when convenient was the answer. 'Thank you,' I said. I signed on that understanding a year ago and never got the leave. I was determined to get this leave, as my new contract would be for the 'duration' and also because I had had no ordinary leave for twenty months. I stated my case on paper. The ADMS came to see me, and after some sarcastic remarks, said that if I insisted, he would forward the papers to Army Headquarters, but he did not for a moment suppose that anything would come of it. I did insist, and in three days I had my leave warrant.

Chapter 12

Nieuport

On return from leave I was posted to a new division, the 32nd, and eventually found myself with the 90th Field Ambulance at la Panne. The normal staff of an FA consisted of nine MOs and a quartermaster, plus, of course, other ranks. For considerable periods, there was little enough for these men to do, and a number of medical officers complained officially that they were kept hanging about in France, when they might be more useful employed elsewhere. A commission, under the chairmanship of Sir Norman Walker, was appointed to investigate the matter, and a questionnaire was sent out to all MOs. The chief question was, 'How many hours a day do you devote to professional work on average?'

Most MOs stated four hours. I put down two. The CO, anxious to preserve his staff intact, paraded us for the purpose of remonstrance.

'Great heavens,' he said on coming to me, 'you have only put two hours!'

'Yes, sir.'

'What do you mean?'

'That is my honest opinion, sir.'

'Have you ever been MO to a regiment?'

'Yes, sir.'

'Then you would be on duty for twenty-four hours per diem.'

'On duty, sir, but not necessarily working.'

'How do you work out your two hours?'

'Sick parade, one hour. Sanitary inspection, one hour, sir.'

'But what about strafes?'

'Included, on the average, sir.'

'Well, when I was an RMO, what with sick, sanitary, etc., I was kept going all day.'

'I have known days in the line, sir, when there was no sick, and no wounded.'

'Do you intend to stick to this, then?'

'Yes, sir.'

'Then you will be a marked man, and such will have more work thrust upon you.'

'Very good, sir, I shall be glad of something to do.'

He was as good as his word, and detailed me for every possible duty, but bore no malice. A Canadian in the division was in a greater disgrace. He put down one hour, and on remonstrance, detailed his answer, starting with base hospital four hours, and ending with FA half an hour!

One day I took the men to bathe. Turing left at the sea front (as ordered) I marched the men along the shore, away from the town. We came to a stake with the inscription: 'No bathing beyond this point.' I took this to refer to the town side, and halted the men some fifty yards farther on. There were only two houses at this point, and one was empty. The men, who were devoid of bathing costumes, had just splashed into the sea, when a military policeman galloped furiously up. Was I in charge of the party?

'Yes.'

'Your men can't bathe here, sir.'

'Look for yourself,' I said, 'they are bathing.'

'Well, you are in front of the Queen's residence.'

And it was so, but nothing could be done about it. As I pointed out to him, the men must return for their clothes. At that he galloped off, and I can only hope that the Queen was not unduly shocked!

Relief work took me into the Redan at Nieuport, with the Dorsets. The Redan was a kind of island territory, cut off from the rest of the line by the River Yser. This was crossed by a double row of duckboards, wired together, and floating on barrels, called Putney Bridge. When the tide was in, the 'bridge' was approximately level with the banks. When the tide was out, the boards sagged down the bank some fifteen feet to the water's edge. The river was about fifty yards wide, and every day the bridge was broken by shell fire, the wretched REs having continually to go out and repair it. It may be imagined with what difficulty one got a stretcher case across at night! Many men were drowned. A man heavily laden, with ration bags slung over his shoulders, crossing in the dark, would come to a point where the duck-boards had been blown away,

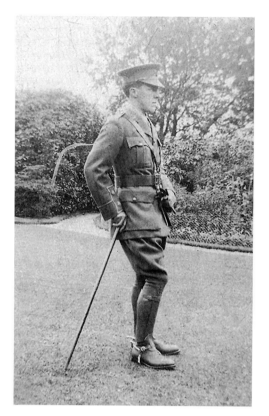

Right: **Figure 1.** Photograph of Captain Harry Gordon Parker, in full dress uniform, taken at the family House, Park Nook, Gosforth, Cumbria. *(Image courtesy of C. Cooper)*

Below: **Figure 2.** University of Edinburgh Roll of Honour, Record of Service, 1914-1918. Captain Harry Gordon Parker is listed fourth from the bottom. *(National Library of Scotland. Public Domain)*

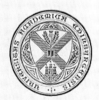

UNIVERSITY OF EDINBURGH

ROLL OF HONOUR

1914—1919

EDINBURGH

Printed and Published for the University by

OLIVER AND BOYD, TWEEDDALE COURT

LONDON: 33 PATERNOSTER ROW, E.C.

1921

Record of War Service

PARHAM, WILLIAM MASKELYNE.
Merchant Taylors' School, London. M.B., C.M. 1889; M.D. 1902. Civil Surgeon, South Africa, 1900-2. R.A.M.C., Captain Sept. 1915; Major Dec. 1915. 47th Casualty Clearing Station, France. Invalided home 1917.

PARIS, GODFREY ANTHONY.
Student of Medicine, 1911-17; M.B., Ch.B. 1916. O.T.C. Medical, Nov. 1914, Cadet. R.N.V.R., Surgeon-Probationer.

PARIS, JOHN.
George Heriot's School. M.A. 1913. O.T.C. Infantry, Oct. 1910 to May 1914, Cadet. 5th Royal Highlanders (Black Watch) (T.), Private April 1916; L./Corporal May 1916; Sergeant Aug. 1916. 5th Border Regiment (T.), 2nd Lieut. Feb. 1917; Lieut. Aug. 1918.

PARISH, HENRY JAMES.
Perth Academy. Student of Medicine, 1913-18; M.B., Ch.B. (Hons.) 1918. O.T.C. Medical, Feb. 1916 to July 1918, Cadet. R.A.M.C., Lieut. Sept. 1918; Captain Sept. 1919. 18th Stationary Hospital, Tiflis, the Black Sea.

PARK, GEORGE WILLIAMSON.
Royal High School; First XV. and XI. M.B., C.M. 1893; B.Sc. (P.H.) 1896. Chief Censor, Penang, 1914. Penang Volunteers, Sergeant 1916-17. Bowhill Auxiliary R.C. Hospital, Selkirk, 1918.

PARK, ROBERT.
Royal High School. M.B., Ch.B. 1911; M.D. 1914. R.A.M.C., Lieut. May 1915; Captain May 1916. France 1915-17. Wounded at Somme 1916. Torpedoed 1917.

PARK, THOMAS GLOVER.
Student of Medicine, 1902-6. R.N.V.R., Sub-Lieut.

PARKER, HARRY GORDON.
Durham School. M.B., Ch.B. 1912. Royal Navy, Temp. Surgeon Sept. 1914. R.A.M.C., Temp. Lieut. Aug. 1915; Captain Aug. 1916. France and The Rhine (three years). Field Ambulance. 51st Manchester Regiment.

PARKER, HERBERT GEORGE.
Student of Medicine. F.R.C.S. (Edin.) 1897. R.A.M.C. (T.), 1901; Lieut.-Col. Nov. 1912. Egypt and Gallipoli. 1st Field Ambulance, Lancashire Division. Nell Lane Military Hospital, Manchester.

PARKER, JAMES SMITH.
Student of Arts and Science, 1910-15; M.A. (Hons. Maths.) 1915; B.Sc. School-master. R.E. (Special Brigade), 4th Battn., Corporal July 1915. Munitions, 1916-19.

PARKER, ROBERT OVEREND.
Dundee High School; Athletics. Student of Science, 1917-19. O.T.C. Engineers, March to Oct. 1918, Cadet. R.E., Officer Cadet Nov. 1918.

2 N 2

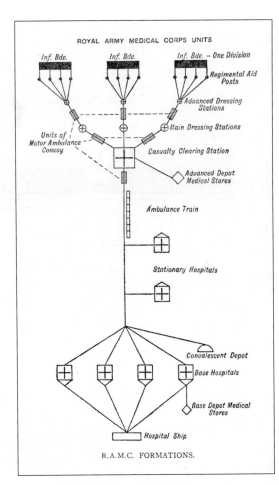

ROYAL ARMY MEDICAL CORPS UNITS

Inf. Bde.   Inf. Bde.   Inf. Bde. – One Division

Regimental Aid Posts

Advanced Dressing Stations

Units of Motor Ambulance Convoy

Main Dressing Stations

Casualty Clearing Station

Advanced Depot Medical Stores

Ambulance Train

Stationary Hospitals

Convalescent Depot

Base Hospitals

Base Depot Medical Stores

Hospital Ship

R.A.M.C. FORMATIONS.

Left: **Figure 3.** Royal Army Medical Corps diagram of the chain of casualty evacuation. *(Wellcome Collection Attribution 4.0 International CC BY 4.0)*

Below: **Figure 4.** Grey wash drawing of Royal Army Medical Corps working in the trenches after a severe engagement. Fortunio Matania. *(Wellcome Collection Attribution 4.0 International CC BY 4.0)*

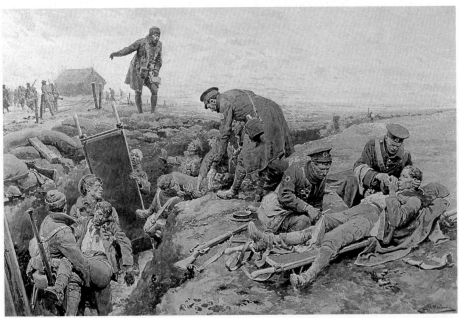

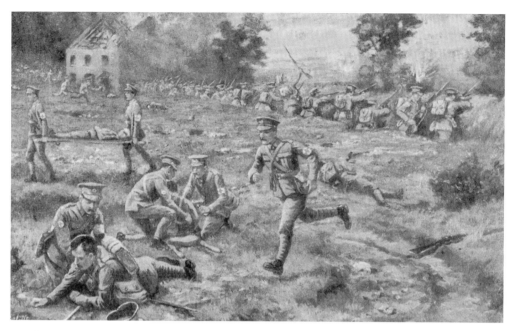

Figure 5. Postcard of Royal Army Medical Corps administering aid to the wounded. Raphael Tuck and Sons. *(Wellcome Collection Attribution 4.0 International CC BY 4.0)*

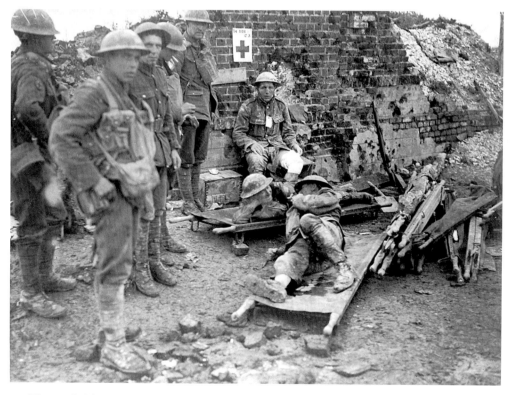

Figure 6. First World War Regimental Aid Post. *(Wellcome Collection First World War Regimental Aid Post)*

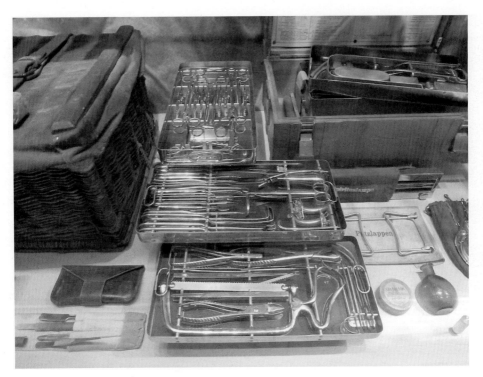

Figure 7. Medical Officers equipment, Memorial Museum, Passchendaele. *(ThruTheseLines Attribution 4.0 International CC BY 4.0)*

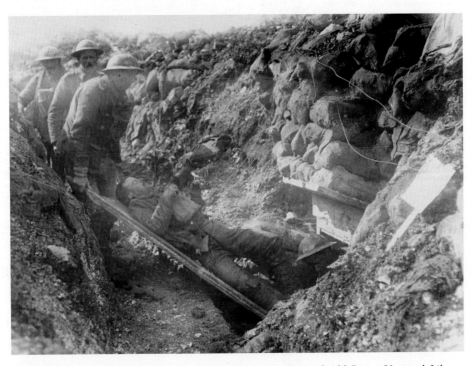

Figure 8. Stretcher Bearers lifting a casualty into a Regimental Aid Post. *(National Library of Scotland. Attribution 4.0 International CC BY 4.0)*

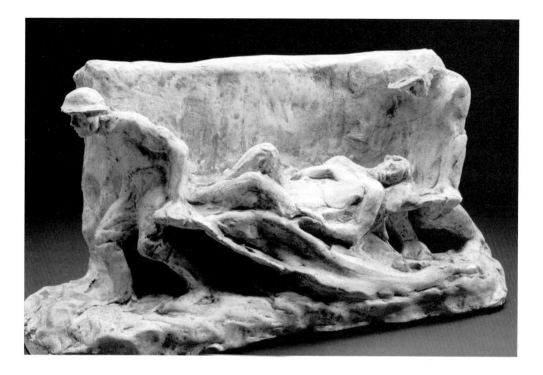

Above: **Figure 9.** Plaster plaque of stretcher bearers carrying wounded soldier 1914-1920 Science Museum, London. *(Wellcome Collection Attribution 4.0 International CC BY 4.0)*

Right: **Figure 10.** Bandaging the wounded in the field. *(Wellcome Collection Attribution 4.0 International CC BY 4.0)*

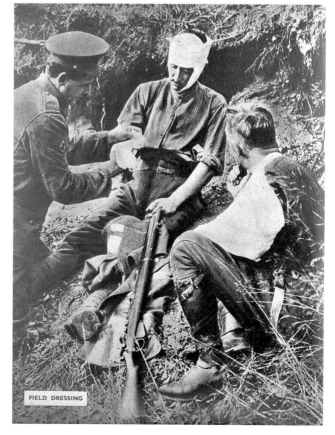

FIELD DRESSING

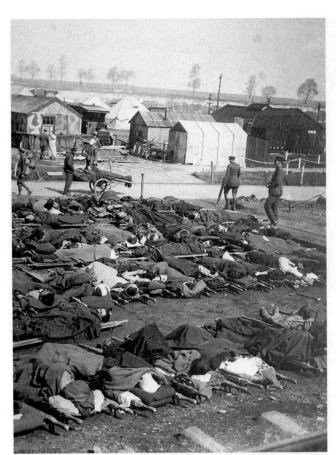

Figure 11. German and British wounded soldiers waiting to be evacuated, Grevillers, Bapume. *(Wellcome Collection L0009184 Attribution 4.0 International CC BY 4.0)*

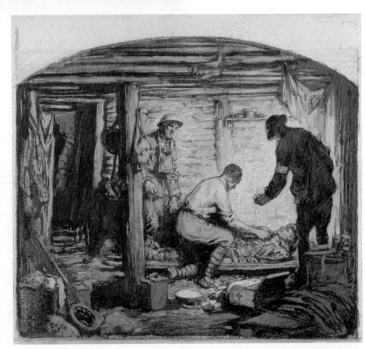

Figure 12. Coloured charcoal drawing depicting a physician attending to a soldier in the trenches. *(Wellcome Collection No. 2436i Public Domain Mark)*

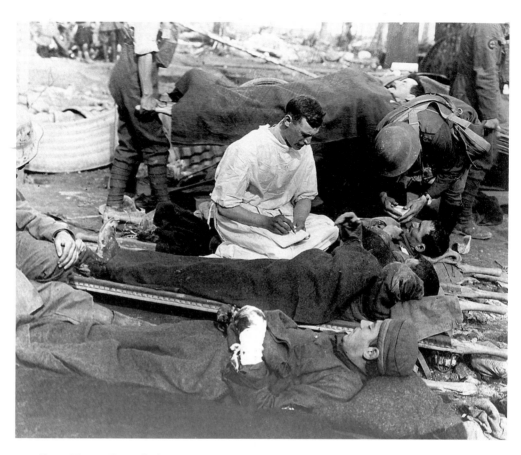

Above: **Figure 13.** Medical Officer noting down a wounded soldier's details at a collection point. *(Wellcome Collection Attribution 4.0 International CC BY 4.0)*

Right: **Figure 14.** Royal Army Medical Corps at Monchy dressing station, France. *(Rijksmuseum, Amsterdam RP-F-F06305 CCO.1.0 Universal Public Domain Dedication)*

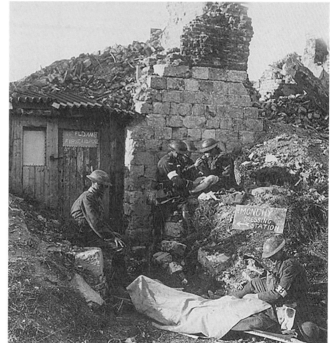

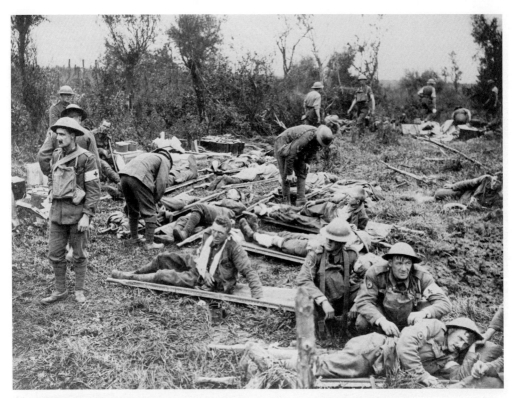

Figure 15. Advance Dressing Station in the field, France. *(Wellcome Collection Attribution 4.0 International CC BY 4.0)*

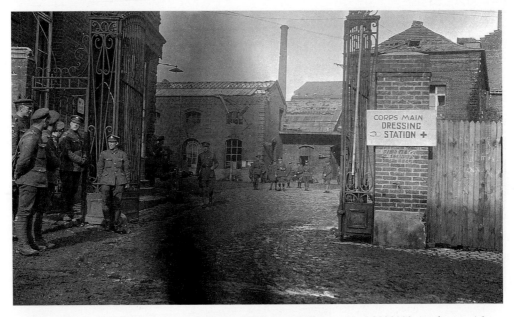

Figure 16. First World War dressing station. *(Wellcome Collection No L0009298 Attribution 4.0 International CC BY 4.0)*

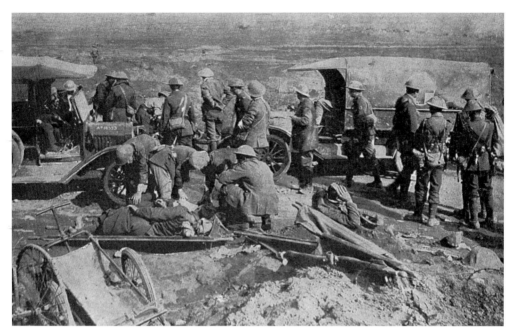

Figure 17. First aid on the battlefield at Advance Dressing Station on the Somme front. *(Wellcome Collection Attribution 4.0 International CC BY 4.0)*

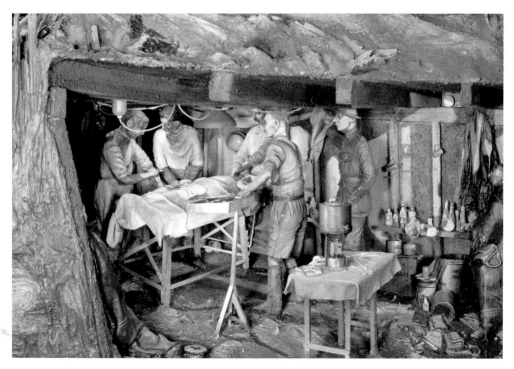

Figure 18. Diorama of Western Front dressing station. Science Museum, London. *(Wellcome Collection Attribution 4.0 International CC BY 4.0)*

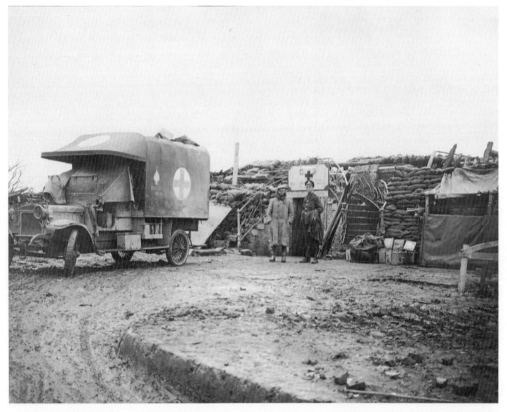

Figure 19. Casualty Clearing Station on the Western Front. *(National Library of Scotland Attribution 4.0 International CC BY 4.0)*

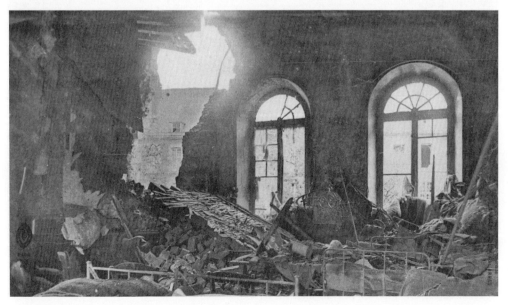

Figure 20. Remains of Hospital St Jean, Arras after heavy shelling by the Germans. *(CC BY 4.0 Public Domain)*

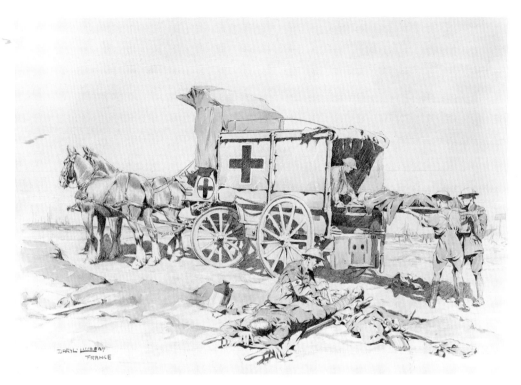

Figure 21. Grey wash drawing of horse ambulance at Ypres by Sir D Lindsay. *(Wellcome Collection Attribution 4.0 International CC BY 4.0)*

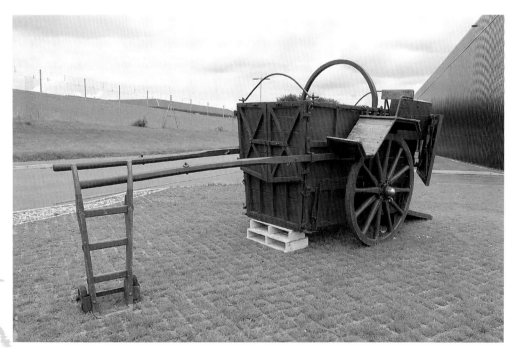

Figure 22. Mock-up of First World War horse drawn ambulance. Royal Logistic Corps Museum. *(G. Cornelius Attribution 4.0 International CC BY 4.0)*

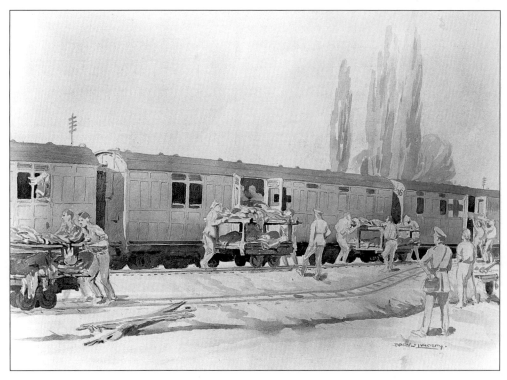

Figure 23. Grey wash drawing of Red Cross ambulance train loading up the wounded at a Casualty Clearing Station. D. Lindsay. *(Wellcome Collection Attribution 4.0 International CC BY 4.0)*

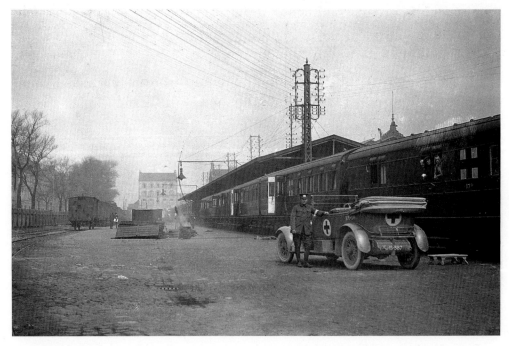

Figure 24. First World War Ambulance Train. *(Wellcome Collection Attribution 4.0 International CC BY 4.0)*

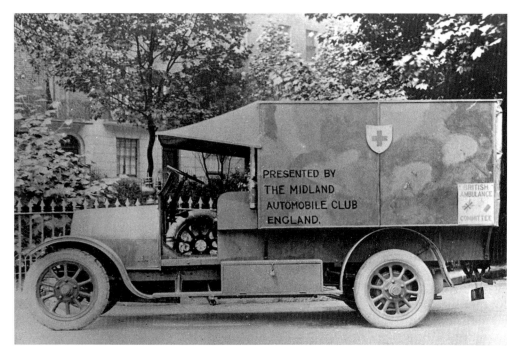

Figure 25. First World War Motor Ambulance. *(Wellcome Collection Attribution 4.0 International CC BY 4.0)*

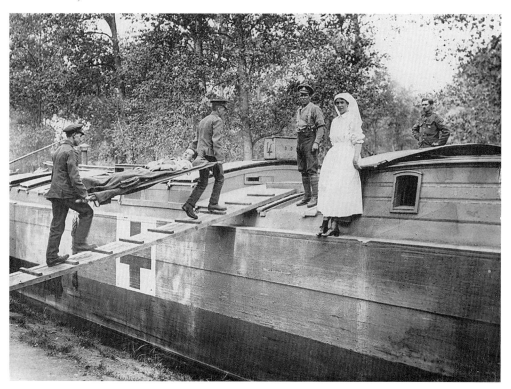

Figure 26. Patients carried aboard a hospital barge on the Western Front. *(Dutch National Archives. CCC 1.0 Public Domain Dedication)*

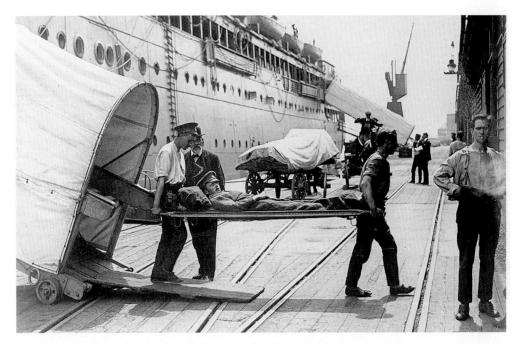

Figure 27. Wounded being carried from a British hospital ship. *(Wellcome Collection Attribution 4.0 International CC BY 4.0)*

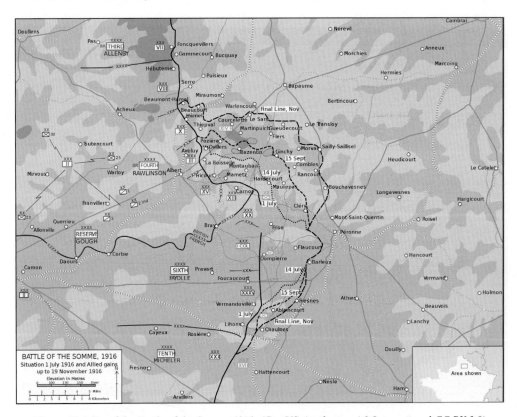

Figure 28. Map of the Battle of the Somme 1916. *(GiroUS Attribution 4.0 International CC BY 3.0)*

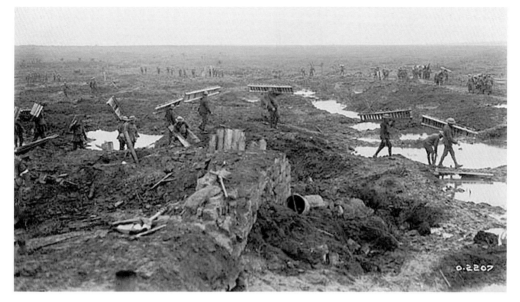

Figure 29. Soldiers carrying duckboards across the mud-filled landscape of Passchendaele by W. Rider. *(Image Library and Archives, Canada. Public Domain Mark)*

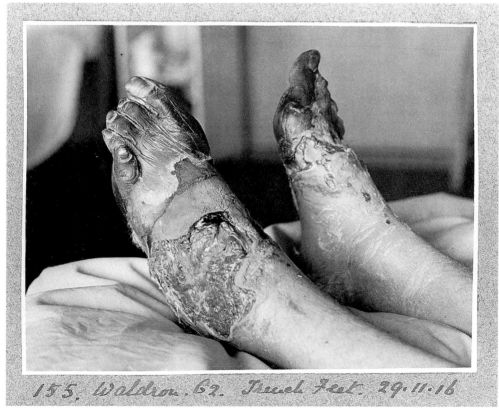

Figure 30. Trench Feet Image No 155 King George Military Hospital. *(Wellcome Collection CMACRAMC 760/L0025834 Attribution 4.0 International CC BY 4.0)*

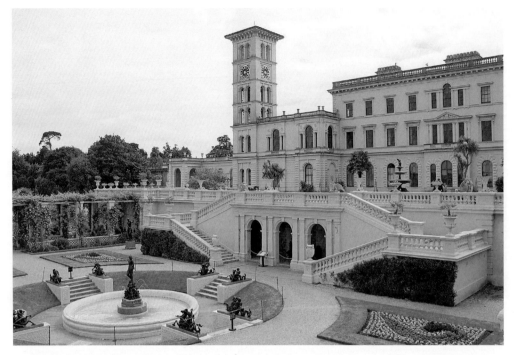

Figure 31. Osbourne House, Queen Victoria's family retreat, Isle of Wight. Utilised as a convalescence home for military officers during the First World War. *(Sulcasmo Attribution 4.0 International CC BY 4.0)*

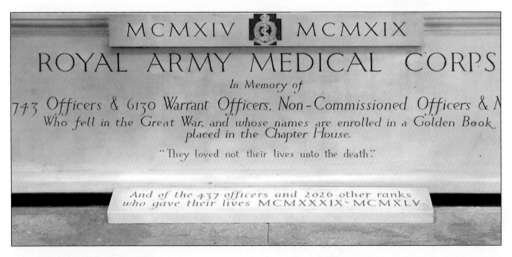

Figure 32. Commemoration dedicated to the Royal Army Medical Corps, Westminster Abbey. *(Authors Own Photograph)*

leaving the wire intact. PLOP! And he was seen no more, till the body was washed up by the tide.

A huge concrete building, known as the Rubber House, stood on the bank, and beyond this were a line of earthworks, like railway embankments, which we called the ramparts. My aid post was a dug-out in the ramparts. The fifty-yard-wide space, between the rampart and the river, was consistently shelled. One night eleven Borders were knocked out at the aid post door buy a single whizz-bang.

A persistent attack of toothache and earache did not increase the pleasure of this trip! The Dorsets came out, and still on relief work, I went in again with the 17th HLI – to the same filthy spot. An attack of dysentery made frequent excursions into the open inevitable. Dashing out to the latrine one night, I heard 'one coming' and threw myself flat in the mud. Something white gleamed near me, and I found that I was lying between two dead men, and staring into the waxy face of one!

The division was being withdrawn and the ADMS was showing his opposite number the glories of the sector that he was handing over. In all the splendour of clean clothes, and shiny leggings, they were received by the Canadian (before mentioned).

'We bury our refuse on waste ground,' said the ADMS, 'and then plant a stake, to show that the ground is foul. Isn't that so, Captain------- ?'

'Yes, sir.'

'Perhaps we should show the Colonel some of these stakes.'

'I can't, sir,' said Canada bluntly.

'What do you mean – can't?' said the ADMS, bridling.

'Because, whenever we put a stake in, a shell blows it out, and the refuse with it, as a rule.'

'Hum! Ah! These ramparts are honeycombed with dug-outs. Excellent billets for the men!'

'Perhaps you would care to inspect them, Sir?' said Canada.

The Canadian led the way, taking them through good dug-outs first. Then turning a corner and twisting through the maze, until they had lost their bearings, took them to a lower level. The ground became damp, water came over their boots, and the ADMS, seeing a streak of light, suggested that they might now conveniently leave the tunnel.

'Oh, sir!' said the guide in horrified tones, 'It's impossible! To go out here is certain death!'

The crash of a shell seemed to confirm his words, and he led them remorselessly on, until the water reached above their knees. Then he led them out at the most dangerous point that he could think of.

'Show me that excellent Aid-Post – Fisher Post, said ADMS, shaking his wet breeches.

'There, sir,' said Canada, pointing to a crumpled heap of masonry.

'I want FISHER POST,' said the ADMS testily.

'That's the only Fisher Post I know of in these parts, sir. And now, sir, if you will excuse me, I must be getting back to my own aid post. If you want to return to the RA, you will have to go round by C Bridge, higher up the river.'

And as soon as their backs were turned, he scampered back to his aid post, ignoring the tunnel. What the ADMS said to the ADMS subsequently I, unfortunately, do not know!

Re-joining the FA, at the CRS at Zudycote, I found one marquee full of cases of rheumatism and trench fever. The men were on stretchers laid on the ground. There were pools of water on the ground, and in some cases the sag of the canvas, under the men's buttocks, within an inch of water. The CO was away, and I sent the whole of the cases on down the line. No doubt this spoiled his batting average, so it was not surprising that I was found a job with the 15th HLI, not this time out of the line unfortunately. Re-joining the RA, it fell to my lot as the youngest MO, to take them for a cross-country run. Collecting them outside, I said: 'We will run round those two windmills,' and led them off at a smart trot, but I had sadly misjudged the distance of those two windmills. When you are on the wrong side of thirty, it is some job taking lads of eighteen to twenty for a run! Still, I did the course, and finished somewhere in the first ten – but never again! About this time, I made contact once more with the 17th Lancashire Fusiliers. Hodgkin's still had his job, and Corporal Holmes' grin was as wide as ever, but poor Crook had fallen to the level of sanitary man, 'cos he couldn't hear the MO!'

Chapter 13

The Manchesters' Passchendaele

Next, I was sent as a relief to the 2nd Battalion the Manchester Regiment, and this became a permanency, as their MO had joined the regulars, and in consequence had been sent to the base. Incidentally, I never saw a regular MO in the front line. I remained with the 2nd Manchester Regiment for the duration. They were a fine lot of lads, and I was proud to be their MO. I joined them at Tunnelling Camp, behind the Ypres sector. The CO's name was Vaughan. After snarling at me at our first encounter, he ever after treated me with the greatest kindness – why I never understood.

We went into the line at Passchendaele. My aid post was pill-box No. 83, and though it sank into the mud up to the loopholes, it was one of the few dry ones. When I visited HQ and found their pill-box held some eighteen inches of black water, over which a floor of duckboards on supports had been laid, so reducing the headroom that one could not sit upright, I feared that the CO would pinch mine as soon as he knew of it. Fortunately, it turned out to be a yard or two outside the battalion area, having been conceded by the artillery for use as an aid post only. Floor space was about 7ft by 6ft; head-room just over 5ft; walls 3½ ft. thick; roof 5ft thick, pierced at the end away from the door by an observation shaft. The top of the doorway was about level with the mud. The inner ends of the loopholes made useful shelves, one of which was used for cooking purposes. To reach the post from Ypres, one had to walk some five or six kilometres along a duckboard track, laid on the mud. The enemy had the track well taped, but it was necessary to keep to it or sink in the mud. The same mud, however, afforded a measure of protection, as the shells sank deeply into it. In frosty weather, there was more danger from splinters, but you could walk wide of the track, and take shelter in shell holes. Normally our chief difficulty was water. Round us there was plenty, but each shell hole had its dead man or dead mule. Water was brought from Ypres in petrol tins. Petrol mixed with water gives a flavour of onions, and when the water had also been chlorinated, you have a really foul mixture to make tea with. The only thing to do was to lace the cup with a lot of rum.

On our first tour of the sector we were short of food also, our ration bag having failed to arrive. We dug some bully beef out of the mud, but would have been practically destitute had we not seen the RAMC squad (who had a lean-to outside the pillbox) about to throw away a chunk of bacon. They said that they could not cook it – well, we could – and from Monday to Saturday, with economy, we lived on that bacon, together with a dozen eggs, that a truly noble batman went back to Poperinghe for, a journey of nearly eighteen kilometres.

The trenches were held under terrible conditions. It snowed and thawed, and the men stamped about in the slush all day. At night, if the ground was firm enough, they would clamber out and run about on the top, chancing the bursts of fire. I was determined to have some source of heat in the pill-box. We cleared the observation shaft, placed a well-perforated petrol tin on two bricks and lit a wood fire. The smoke had to ascend some three-and-a-half feet to the base of the shaft and at first the place was full of smoke. As the shaft got warm it drew better, and presently by sitting on the floor we were able to keep our heads out of the smoke. Later, a blanket hung in the doorway at the proper angle, made things better still. We camouflaged the top of the 'chimney' with a broken stretcher. It must have been the only fire for miles around, and I believed it saved many lives. Wounded would be brought in by the stretcher-bearers, in a half-frozen condition. Having attended to their wounds, we would put them on a stretcher on the floor, out of the smoke, well covered with blankets, drop the curtains, give them hot tea, and keep them there until thoroughly warmed.

Months later I read an article on proposed methods of rechauffment in the forward areas, but this dealt with a system of lamps and trestle tables in a field ambulance. On the Saturday rations arrived for us from three different sources. We gorged on Sunday, and being relieved next morning, left the remainder for the incoming party. Coming out, I slipped off the track and got stuck in the mud for some time, in a very unhealthy spot.

perhaps I should have been called sooner. He lay on the wire bed, his fair hair lying lank across his damp forehead, and in the artificial light he looked frailer than ever. He opened his eyes and looked at me with a kind of fearful dread.

Temperature 102. My duty was obvious!

'You are due for leave,' I said, 'where is your warrant?'

'I won't tell you,' he said, sulkily.

'Come on,' I said. 'Let me see it.'

'You shan't have it,' he cried, his voice rising hysterically.

'Look here J.,' I said, 'you know that I can stop your leave by one word. I only want to look at your warrant. You shall have it back.'

He handed it over, and I saw that he had forty-eight hours to go. Prescribing some treatment, I went out, and enquired as to what men were due for leave. Fortunately, Lesty, one of the mess orderlies was going. I spoke to Lesty, and told him, that if Mr. J. went on leave, he was to act as his batman and look after him on the journey.

Next day J. was considerably better. Sitting down on his bed, I said, 'I will let you go on leave on certain conditions. You must put yourself in Lesty's charge. He will carry all your stuff.'

He nodded.

'When you reach the boat, you must go below at once, and stay there until you reach port.'

Again he nodded.

'One thing more you must promise.' I continued. 'Have a few days at home if you like, but well before your leave is up, you will report sick at the nearest depot.'

'Oh, but I couldn't do that,' he said.

'But you must,' I answered.

'But (in distress), it's such a rotten thing – reporting sick – on leave.'

'Listen,' I said. 'You are not strong enough for this beastly life out here. That's not your fault. You've done your bit for months – more than any hefty man at home. It's your mothering turn now.'

We looked at each other in silence. 'Is that your last word?'

'Those are my terms.'

He got home safely; kept to his word and the battalion knew him no more. A very unmilitary proceeding, no doubt, but as Colonel Robertson once said, 'We shall never make a soldier of a doc.'

In February, a raid was made from a place called Ajax House, for the purpose of dealing with a troublesome machine gun. It was the only obvious successful raid that I knew of. A hundred men went over, a promise being made that a sum of cash and fourteen days' leave would be given to each of the two men who did best in the action. Two machine guns and eight prisoners were captured and eighteen shoulder-straps from dead Germans were brought in, while it was known that many more of the enemy had been killed. Part of the Report to Brigade read: '... We captured ... Machine guns ... Our casualties were slight, two killed and seventeen wounded.'

The last sentence made a strange impression upon me. Slight indeed, in proportion to the number engaged, and objectives gained, but what of the two homes that would receive the fatal telegram? It does not do to ponder on such things at the front.

At this time we had in the battalion a man named Sirrett. About two years previously, he was on the point of going on leave, when his company HQ was burnt out. He proceeded on leave, well knowing that all the records had been destroyed. Once at home, he destroyed his uniform and all his military effects, got a job on munitions, and actually obtained a silver protection badge. Being young and healthy, he next took unto himself, not a wife, but a lady friend. Then one night in his cups, stung no doubt by some taunt, he boasted that he was actually in the army and had been to France. Still all went well, until he quarrelled with his lady friend. She gave him away.

Taken back to France, he was tried, and as a defence challenged the court to prove he had ever belonged to the regiment. A number of officers and NCOs had fallen during his absence, but there were many who recognised him perfectly, though none were willing to say so. He was sentenced to death, but instead of being confirmed, the sentence was altered to a term of imprisonment, to be served after the war. Sirrett greatly distinguished himself during the raid, drew the money and fourteens days' leave, had his sentence wiped out, and also got the MM.

Chapter 14

Trench Feet a Crime

At Gambetta my normal aid post was some distance from the front line, which was held by posts. One evening a man reported with trench feet. He was curable, so we dried his boots and puttees, while the feet were massaged with French powder. When the things were dry, we issued him with a new pair of socks, and marking him 'M. and D.', I sent him back to his company. Sometime later, to my intense disgust, the corporal told me that this man had been given fourteen days' [Field Punishment] No. 1 for reporting sick *without a cause*. Worse still, it was too late to take any action, as he had already served the sentence. Thus he was punished for doing his obvious duty in reporting sick, and *preventing him from becoming a casualty*. Punishment is only applicable when a man is marked 'D'.

To have trench feet was at the time practically a crime, and a battalion with a high percentage was frowned upon. I managed to camouflage our numbers, by arranging that slight cases remained with the percentage of strength left out of the line on the next tour. On one occasion my average was spoilt by an interfering person, who, wanting the men for a fatigue, and finding them unable to do it, had all of them sent to hospital. Treatment was mainly by massage with a camphorated French powder. There was a great shortage of this. As a supply for the whole battalion, I would receive about as much as could be held with both hands cupped. Company officers would then indent on me, and be furious when they got about two ounces of their share.

While at Arneke someone in authority had a bright idea, and all the MOs were circularised to the effect that they were to provide each man with a Gold Flake cigarette tin full of the powder, for use as necessary. I calculated that I would need about one and a half cwt [hundredweight], and much doubting whether such an amount existed in the whole BEF, at once wrote out the following indent.

Please supply:

(A) Powder, Foot, French, cwt. 1½.
(B) Tins, Cigarette, Gold Flake, 1,000.

I gave this to the corporal, who much perturbed at such audacity, was shortly heard bewailing, 'He'll be shot! He'll be shot!'

'Who will be shot?' asked someone.

'The MO,' said the wretched corporal. 'Look what he's given me!'

But I never heard another word about the matter. To act dumb, and obey the last order to the letter, was often the way out of an awkward situation.

Orders had been given that foot treatment (preventative and curative) must be carried out when the battalions were out at rest. In this connection we worked a good stunt when at Hospital Farm. We had got wind of an inspection re foot treatment, and our intelligence service had been equal to discovering the day, and probable time of the same. A Nissen hut was cleared, and seats placed down each side, and across the end, with a table in the middle. As the hour approached, a platoon of men was paraded outside the hut. Half a dozen men were placed on the seats along the right side of the hut, and told to remove their footgear. Stretcher-bearers then entered with bowls of hot water, and nail brushes, and proceeded to cleanse the feet and nails with special soap. The first two men washed, were then transferred to the bench at the end of the hut where battalion chiropodists paired their talons. After chiropody, they were moved around to the left-hand benches where their feet were dried, and vigorously massaged with French powder.

Corporal Jefferies stood in the centre doling out soap and powder, controlling the queue, and roaring encouragement to the stretcher-bearers. The show was in full swing when a scout announced that staff cars were approaching. Activity was doubled as a number of gorgeous persons descended from the cars – the DDMS, the ADMS, and an odd general or two. They were received with great respect, and escorted to the hut, where they saw the men 'before and after using your soap,' and in process of ablution and pedicure. Then, expressing themselves delighted with the excellence of the arrangements, they departed in pomp. As soon as they were out of sight, the whole show was closed down – indeed, we had not enough powder and soap to keep it going for more than half an hour. Later on, 'Pedicuria' were established behind the line, and we were relived of responsibility.

At Arneke, a company of WAACs was billeted quite near us. We left this place in the small hours of the morning but the band and the men kicked up such a row when passing the WAACs' billets, that the WAACs stampeded after the battalion, and rushing to the station, delayed the train by clambering on the footboards and hanging out of the windows. There was pandemonium for a time, but good humour and a good sense prevailed, and at length we got a move on.

Conditions at Passchendaele were, I think, the worst that I ever experienced. One night, struggling over the duckboards in the dark, I said to the corporal (who had been out from the beginning), 'Well, I suppose it was worse than this in '14.'

'Don't you believe it, sir,' he answered promptly. 'In '14 there was food to be scrounged, houses to go into and walls to hide behind. Here, we might as well be walking on a billiard table.'

At Easter we were suddenly rushed on south, and after an all-night journey, during which the train was shelled, detrained early on Good Friday at a place the name of which I have forgotten. One company remained to detrain the laden transport, which they accomplished in twenty minutes at a cost of one broken leg, and one man killed. A march, which only ended long after dark, brought us to Adinfer, a position about seven miles east of Arras, where we relieved the Irish Guards. Colonel Vaughan got a brigade soon after this. The man who succeeded him only lasted three weeks. He was succeeded by Colonel Robertson, who came from the Staffords. He was very young for a battalion commander, but no battalion could have wished for a better CO.

Shortly after this, we had notable reinforcement in the person of Major Neville Marshall VC, late of the Irish Guards. He was an imposing personality, with a huge chest plastered with ribbons, and nine wound stripes on his sleeve. A martinet, he struck fear into all hearts, and the moment we were out of the line he insisted on spit and polish, and gruelling drills, though it was the first rest that the men had had for seven weeks. At first he was universally hated. It did not trouble him. One day he told the parade what they were thinking.

'You are thinking,' he said, 'we'll shoot that blighter as soon as we get into action with him. Well,' he continued, turning his broad back to them, 'here's your mark. I shall be in front of you – not behind!' He was as good as his word, and when they had been in action with him, the men worshipped him. I can only say here that he was the finest soldier, and the bravest man, that I ever had the honour to meet. Relieved by the 1st Grenadier Guards, we moved by light railway to la Bezique, passing through orchards and fields of poppies.

We rested at Berneville, billeted in a large wood, with a big farm as BHQ. Sick parade was at 7 a.m., men's breakfasts being 8 a.m. The average officer broke his fast about 8.45. I was punctually on parade on the first morning but did not see the fun of getting up so much earlier than the youngest subaltern. The Guards, who had just left the place, had had two hundred cases of influenza. After parade I wrote the following chit:

From MO I/C 2nd Battalion Manchester Regiment
To OC 2nd Battalion Manchester Regiment

Sir:
I have the honour to observe that sick parade has been ordered for 7.00 hours. This is not altogether satisfactory from a medical point of view. There is an epidemic of influenza. If sick men are congregated in the early morning before being fed, those who have not got influenza will, by reason of being below par, through not having their morning meal, be likely to contract the infection from those who already have the disease. In this way the epidemic may reach alarming proportions in the battalion. I have the honour to suggest, sir:

(1) That breakfasts be earlier.
(2) That sick parade be held later.

I have the honour to be, sir

Your obedient servant,

Entering the mess later, I found the CO and the adjutant together. My chit lay on the table.

'You old scheming devil,' said the C.O. with a twinkle in his eye.

'Of course, we shall take no notice of this, sir,' said the adjutant, indicating the paper.

'Oh yes, we must,' said the CO. 'That is Medical Advice.'

The discomfited adjutant was compelled to alter the time of sick parade to 9 a.m. I gave the 'Excused Duty' to all men with the slightest temperature, and made the whole parade gargle each morning. We had less than a score of cases of influenza in the battalion, and very few of them had to be evacuated. The alteration in time made no difference to the size of the parade – I knew the men, and they knew me – but bitterness remained in the adjutant's soul.

A soccer match was arranged, Officers v. NCOs. At the last moment I was warned to play in place of the adjutant. Running on to the field late, I had kicked the ball twice, and had been knocked down once, when a great blast on the whistle warned us to fall in ready to move. All scampered to their stations, and in twenty minutes the whole battalion was standing on the road all limbered up, waiting to move forward, and wondering where Jerry had broken through. Then we were ordered back to our quarters. It was just a little stunt on the part of the major. I understood then why the adjutant had stood down from the team at the last moment.

We returned to the line in the Boiry-au-Mare sector, and about this time we commenced a new stunt in the war against the louse. The stretcher-bearers were armed with flat irons, and when a platoon went into the baths, the bearers went with them. The men's clothes were given to the stretcher-bearers, and while the men were in the bath, the bearers ran their hot irons along the seams of the clothing, to kill the lice, and in the hope of destroying at least a percentage of the eggs. When possible, the men were given a clean change of underclothing on emerging from the bath.

As a result of experience gained at Arras and in other places, in cases of fractured femur, it was decided to supply Thomas's Splints to RMOs. This splint resembled a gigantic hairpin, the wide end of which was encircled by a padded leather ring. The ring was slipped over the foot and pushed up to the groin. Extension was then made on the limb, by tying bandages round the ankle, and fixing the other end of the bandage to the narrow angle of the splint. Bandages or other material, passing from rod to rod below the leg, formed a cradle for the limb. The whole splint was now slung from a suspension bar, an affair like a soccer goal-post, which was clamped onto the stretcher-poles at the right point. The whole limb thus swung easily from the hip joint with each movement of the stretcher. A number of minor adjustments afforded scope to the ingenuity of the MO.

A number of MOs protested that it would be impossible to apply this splint in a shell hole. Actually it was possible to apply it under almost any conditions provided you were sufficiently determined. Three such splints were allotted to each RMO, and bearers who took a case down were charged with the duty of bringing another splint back to replace that on a patient. The arrangement worked admirably and after this innovation the mortality in cases of fractured femur fell by fifty per cent. Apart from that, the invariable expression of gratitude on the part of the patient after the splint had been fixed made any difficulty of applications well worthwhile.

There were some MOs who left all the manual work to their orderlies, contenting themselves with signing the evacuation tally. I do not understand the mentality of a man who could deny such surgical skills as he might possess to men in pain. I don't say that I myself got up for every small scratch that came in the night, but I did get up for every fracture.

The problem of manpower had, of course, become acute before this date, and all special departments were asked to reduce their numbers. I had eight stretcher-bearers in each company, the leader of each squad having a lance stripe. Four men assisted me in the aid post, including the medical corporal and my batman, Walter Bennett. I submitted a scheme by which the company bearers would be reduced to five per company, but much to my relief the CO told me that he would prefer I stick to my original number, saying that he would show the extra men as rifles in his return. What a difference from 1915, when, with more men available than could be properly equipped, I had to beg my normal personnel.

Sometime in July we were sent to Proven, behind Pop, for a real rest. Here I had a clash with the major. In his gingering up of the battalion he interfered with practically everybody. One day I learned that he had given a man a dose of medicine. This got my goat and I went in search of him. We met in the mess.

'I want to see you, sir,' I said abruptly.

'Yes, doc.,' said the major, producing his really charming smile.

'You have given a man medicine. You have no right to do so.'

Instead of bellowing with rage as one might have expected of a man who got all his own way, and brooked opposition from none, he sat down quietly and looked at me.

'But------, ' he began.

'I am the Medical Officer of this battalion, not you,' I continued. 'You may be a wonderful man, but you can't do everyone's job.'

'But I only wanted to help.'

'I don't need help. I have a corporal.'

'Really, it was with the best intentions.'

'I have one job to do here, and I can do it.'

'No one doubts it, doc.,' he said. 'Come into my hut and let us talk it over.'

We went into his hut, where he reiterated his benevolent intentions.

'But, sir,' I said, 'you are interfering with discipline.'

'Ah, doctor,' he said, smiling once more. 'Now we are going to agree.'

And so it was. I had never been so rude to a senior officer before, but he bore me no grudge, and shortly afterwards did me a considerable service. How it came to be I will relate.

The adjutant had long nursed a grievance about the time of the sick parade and, one evening in the mess, after tea, started to throw his weight about, and get on to me. When I answered him with some spirit, he told me angrily that the mess was not the place to discuss such matters. I at once agreed but reminded him that he had been the first to broach the subject. At this he got into a rage, and after a few threats, said he would make me do sick parade at seven a.m. before I was much older.

'If you wish to be a swine,' I replied, 'you are certainly in a favourable position to carry out the intention.'

He flung out of the mess and within an hour I had a written order to do sick parade at 7 a.m. next morning. I felt resentful and rebellious, and it was here that Major Marshall stepped in, asking me to go with him to the Quartermaster's stores, by lorry to la Panne, early next morning, to try and get some barrels of beer for the men.

'What about sick parade, sir?' I asked.

'Oh, you can do that when you come back. I'll arrange it,' he said.

At la Panne, we were most politely received by Comery, the Commandant, or whatever he was, but he would not part with any beer. Being in no hurry to leave that pleasant spot, we took a stroll along the sands, and I told Comery about the order, and intimated that I felt inclined to ignore it.

'Doc.,' he said, 'I'm a much older soldier than you. Take my advice and do it. The adjutant was on the phone to Brigade last night. He was asking for authority for that order, and got it, so if you don't obey you know what is likely to happen!'

I was on parade in the morning, and noted that the adjutant was also up early! I have no doubt that the Major sent me on the journey to la Panne to get me out of the way, and give me twenty-four hours to think things over. Three days later the order was washed out, and this also, I believe, was the Major's doing.

Chapter 15

The Advance – le Quesnoy

Early in August we went south. On the 8th we commenced to chase the Canadians, first by bus, and then on foot. As we were climbing on the buses, the Major shoved half a cold chicken into my hand, telling me that there was not much chance of getting anything else that day. This is just one example of his kindness – if he thought you meant to do your job. On the 10th we caught up with the Canadians at le Quesnoy, where they were held up, and got into action about 8 a.m. It seemed odd to be strolling into battle over open ground switching the heads of thistles with sticks. The enemy must have been taken somewhat by surprise as most of their shells fell behind us. The CO rode his horse for the first 1,500 yards. I also had mine with me, but used him as a pack horse. The Nobbler, an old pre-war army horse, was almost human, and hopped over trenches with the splints rattling on his back. When the machine-gun fire became a bit thick, we left him in a trench, to be taken back when convenient. The enemy were making a stand, so the advance did not go very far, and I established a permanent aid post in a covered portion of trench.

Here, we soon had plenty of work and were in some difficulty, as the FA did not get in touch with us until 3 p.m. Next morning another brigade attempted to go through us. Had they come at 5 a.m. they might have succeeded, as there was dense fog, As it was, they arrived at the more fashionable hour of 10, when the sun was up and visibility excellent. As such I watched nine of their tanks burst into flames. They had heavy casualties, many of which passed through our post. Major Marshall had jocularly remarked that he was entitled to be the rearmost man in this action, but he was in the thick of the fight, encouraging the men, and promising them good things when the show was over. He had bullets through his tunic and breeches and one lodged in his thigh. Refusing to go to hospital, he had this removed on the field and remained on duty.

The battalion were withdrawn about midnight on the 12th, but my party remained to clean up.

About 7 a.m. we were ready to go, but were uncertain as to whether we could consider ourselves entitled to do so. Then an MO from the FA arrived and, remarking that we looked about done up, took over the post temporarily. After trailing wearily back for two hours, we sighted the battalion resting on some open ground. When we were still some distance off they spotted us. Judge of my surprise, when the adjutant not only came out to meet us, but brought me a cup of tea! Two days later we were scrapping again. It happened thus. We had retired still farther, and were bivouacked in a large field. The adjutant and I were strolling on the grass at some distance from the rest. He was speaking, but I was only giving him half my attention. Presently I heard him say, 'And you and I have got nothing!'

'Got nothing,' I repeated vaguely; then as his meaning penetrated my slow wits, my gorge began to rise.

'Why should we?' I said coldly. 'For my part, I was under cover for a great part of the time.'

'Well,' he said, 'there was getting there, and getting back; and ------ .'

'X,' I said, 'if either you or I deserve the MC for what we did in this last show, then every private in the Battalion deserves the VC.'

He was so annoyed that he scarcely spoke to me for some days.

In this open warfare, we had greater opportunity of picking up material likely to be of use to us. I found that the lids of boxes which had contained German field-gun ammunition made excellent leg splints; made of tin, they were light, strong, and of just the right length and width. Consequently, we kept a sharp lookout for them when advancing. Another thing that was of great use to us was the German serrated bayonet. These weapons, according to propaganda, were supposed to be used for the greater mutilation of victims. As the serrations, which started at the hilt, stopped some five or six inches from the point, this seems scarcely likely. Actually they made very efficient, if somewhat wasteful saws, and this I believe, was the use for which they were invented. I always carried one with me, for the purpose of sawing up wood to make splints.

Also in captured German positions, there [were] nearly always some convenient articles. The stoves which they made had a kidney-shaped opening in the top, which exactly fitted their billy-cans. Halfway down each side of the can itself was a knob, which prevented the vessel from sinking too far into the fire – a great improvement on a mess tin balanced on two bayonets over an open brazier.

Reinforced we went in again at Hevieville at midnight. In the morning we were heavily raided, the enemy leaving nineteen dead in our trenches. When the LFs relieved us, a sturdy looking MO, about twenty-five years of age, took over from me. He seemed very excited on arrival, rushing in and out of the shelter. A few hours later he got a light scratch on the scalp. Instead of reporting himself as a casualty, and awaiting relief, he dashed straight off to the FA and, having had his wound dressed, commenced to babble about the chance of tetanus, meningitis and every other complication. *Sure* enough he did get septic meningitis, and died in a few days. I think he really frightened himself to death.

Two battalions of Lancashire Fusiliers held the line in front of us, but twenty-four hours after relief, we had to send all our companies to reinforce these two units. Gas was being used, and eye cases were crawling back by platoons. There must have been some lack of supervision in fixing the gas-masks, as we had practically no cases, though we lay close behind them. A day later we took over the right of Quarry sector, and next morning the battalion made an attack without artillery support, and succeeded in taking the village of Vermandovillers, and in penetrating to a depth of two miles. Having been up to the limit of the advance, I returned to the Quarry for my aid post staff and there met the divisional general and told him what had happened. He cross-questioned me closely, before going forward to see for himself. I got my aid post party up, and established them in a shelter on the right flank. No further advances could be made until the flanking force came up, so as we were there for the night, I had to have some relay posts between us and the old line.

Returning to the Quarry, I found that a dozen RAMC men had arrived. The sergeant in charge firmly refused to go farther forward, in which he was no doubt right, according to his orders. He offered me four men. As I needed twenty men, I jumped onto the Ford ambulance and went to the AFA two or three miles back. I knew that I could find Captain Rutherford there. He was a pal of mine, and cared nothing for red tape. Rutherford at once promised me all the men that he could spare. As I was about to leave, he said, 'Wait, have some dinner before you go.

The men will start now, and I will send you up to the Quarry by motor ambulance.' This I was glad to do. The ambulance reached the Quarry, not without slipping into a few shell holes. It was now dark, and I had been absent from my post in the line for two or three hours, but I had the right sort of CO and knew that he would understand.

The men were ready and I led them off. Things in the dark looked very different, when seen thus for the first time, and it was not too easy to find the way. Suddenly we were challenged.

'RAMC,' cried several shrill voices behind me. The sentry was unimpressed.

'MR,' I said clearly, 'Medical Officer bringing up bearers.' He gave me the OK but before advancing I turned to the party and said, 'Next time we are challenged, keep your mouths shut. I will answer. Nothing makes the Infantry shoot quicker than a shout of RAMC.'

I posted the squads at intervals of about half a mile, taking the last one on to the aid post. It was then midnight, and having been on the go since 6 a.m. I stretched out on the floor. Sergeant Jefferies (he had been promoted) was saying something about the battalion having retired during my absence.

'Can't help it.'

'But we are in No Man's Land, sir.'

'Don't care. Go to sleep.'

After all these precautions, of course, nothing happened during the night, but one had to be prepared. About 6 a.m. Bennett went to draw rations, and found that the battalion had disappeared. We made a little tea, ate a biscuit apiece, and loading our stuff on to a wheel stretcher, set off with no great certainty as to direction. Fortunately, a mounted staff officer met us, and gave us a point to march on. After walking four or five hours, we saw the battalion halted ahead of is. When we were still some three hundred yards away, they fell in, and moved off. Dinner had gone west as breakfast had done!

On the afternoon of the third day, our cautious advance reached Château Misery, about three kilometres from the Somme. (Relief was impossible, as the two other battalions could only muster about a hundred men each). The Major, who had again been wounded, wanted to take a platoon of men and try to cross the river, but the CO ruled that the men had had enough. Nevertheless, he (the Major) called for three volunteers, at once got them, reached the river, and under fire chalked '2nd MR 29th Aug. 1918' on the bridge, at Cizancourt.

There were huts in the château grounds, with inviting looking bunks, but the CO wisely made us lie in trenches outside the wall. The grounds were shelled next morning. Later in the day, another brigade came up and occupied the huts. The wisdom of our CO was evident when, sometime after midnight, a runner woke me, and gave me a message scrawled on a fragment of a map, directing me to proceed immediately to brigade headquarters. Fortunately, I was sufficiently awake to retain the guide, but it was soon evident where we were wanted, for 9.2s were crashing in the château grounds. We reached the Lodge, which was intact, and in the cellar found a collection of brigade personnel including a staff officer shivering in pyjamas, and wondering if he might rush upstairs and get his British warm.

There were plenty of casualties in the grounds. While attending to them word reached me that a number of wounded were collected in a tunnel under the ruined château. I went to the tunnel, ordering that other wounded were to be brought to me there. Here we worked for two or three hours by the light of two guttering candles stuck in the wall. There were wooden bunks in the tunnels, and soon I wanted splints. A word was enough for Sergeant Jefferies to start kicking the nearest bunk to pieces. Up sat an indignant officer, to enquire what the devil he meant.

'Medical Officer's orders,' said the Sergeant, aiming another kick. 'We need splints.'

To the officer's credit he vacated the bunk without further comment. As I bent over one stretcher, another was lifted over my head. This stretcher held a large pool of blood, and as it tilted the blood cascaded down my back. Eventually I stretched my back, and sat down for a moment against the wall. Near me was an officer. We were both in shirt-sleeves and neither recognised the other. Blood had been spilt over the bandages of a case lying before us. The officer said, 'Can't you do something for him?'

'I could and I would,' I replied wearily, 'if he needed it.'

The officer continued to whittle about the case (which was all fixed up) until, getting ratty, I said, 'For heavens' sake let me know something about my own job.'

It was only later that I discovered that he was one of the gilded staff!

During the night the transport had come up, and parked in the orchard. About breakfast time they got it hot. Going to the rescue, we met the Maltese cart dashing down the road, with Pollitt standing on the shafts and driving like Jehu. We arrested it to have spare stretchers thrown off to us. The QM stores had been hit, only one out of ten men left alive, and two poor lads had been killed at the door with leave warrants in their hands! Smith, one of my orderlies, had also been caught. This man had had more than one chance of a safe billet behind the lines. On the previous evening he had returned from hospital at his own request, and not knowing the location of the aid post, had spent the night with the transport. He was blown to pieces before he could leave the lines.

The battalion retired about two kilometres, and we stayed until we had cleared all cases. Searching the place for material, I found several perfectly good stretchers with the canvas wantonly ripped from top to bottom. The battalion remained where they were, until the fall of Peronne enabled them to cross the Somme safely. The weather was fine, and we slept in moss-lined shell holes of 1916, and experienced some most gorgeous sunsets. Now, in the early days of the war with many willing helpers, and comparatively few wounded, cases sometimes received over-attention. An enthusiastic Red Cross man, or VAD, would spot a casualty, and pounce on him eagerly, so that men would almost flee at the sight of a nurse, giving rise to the story of the man who pleaded, 'Please don't dress my wounds, miss, it's been dressed six times this morning already.'

This is not meant as a gibe at voluntary helpers, or at those who did such splendid service in work to which they were quite unaccustomed. It is only the record of a fact. It occurred to me that if a case could be efficiently put up on the front line, he might be spared the pain and delay of dressings at some of the intermediate posts.

To this end I could put in a great amount of time and labour, in fixing splints and arranging dressings at the RAP which I fear at times taxed the patience of my sergeant who, however, was much too good a soldier to betray his feelings. My hope was that the cases might perhaps travel as far as the CCS without further interference. We had worked in this way for many months without knowing the results of our labours, and I often wondered if our careful adjustments were pulled down, possibly at the AFA. While at rest behind Misery I met a field ambulance MO.

We chatted for a while, and I was leaving him, when he called out, 'Wait – there is something I have been meaning to tell you for a long time. Your cases arrive at the FA in better condition than those of any other unit. In fact, in time of stress, it has become almost an unwritten rule, that cases with your name on the tally, can be sent on without inspection by an MO.'

This was very heartening, but our red letter day was not yet over. Later, I met the ADMS, who congratulated me on having the lowest sick rate in the Division.

'The Manchesters and the umpteenth,' he said, 'are the bright spots of the Division.'

'And the Medical Units, sir,' said an officer standing near him.

'No,' said the ADMS. 'You are far behind the Manchesters.'

These expressions of appreciation, so rare in military life, made everything seem well worthwhile.

We crossed the Somme on 6 September and at one bivouac had a welcome bathe in the River Omignon. Continuing to advance, we reached Villeveque Lake, and here were ordered to make an attack, to take some trenches and part of Holmon Wood. There was to be a barrage at 5 a.m. But the company commanders asked that they might be allowed to make a night attack without artillery. Accordingly, we crept up to Marteville about 11 p.m. Three companies took part in the attack, the fourth remaining in reserve, in a deep railway cutting along the BHQ.

Thirteen is surely my lucky number. I have had the room No. 13, lived in house No. 13, and occupied bed No.13 in hospital, to mention only a few of the occasions on which the number has turned up for me. A year or two ago, I was applying for an appointment in competition with several others. When I heard that the matter was to be decided on the 13th, I told my wife that I had got the job! (I had.) Yet, if I was to select ticket No. 13 in a sweep, I should not expect to win. If, however, I said give me any old number, and then was handed No.13, I should be able to spend the money in advance. Though not actually attached to me, the number appears in the following incident.

The railway cutting was about twenty-five feet deep, and nestling against the foot of the slope were some string sand-bagged shelters, with elephant iron roofs. I chose one as an aid post, the chief consideration being the possibility of getting a loaded stretcher in and out. I was just throwing off my kit when the sergeant said that he had found a better place farther up – a hole which went right into the bank. We moved there, informing the adjutant, who put thirteen men of the reserve company into the shelter. Hardly had we settled our things, when a tremendous explosion seemed to rock the whole embankment. A shell, which at the end of its trajectory, must also have tobogganed down the slope, had struck the corner of the shelter just over the door, flinging the huge sheet of elephant iron right over the opposite bank. The place was a shambles, literally the floor ran with blood. Of the thirteen men, seven were dead and the remainder very badly wounded, those farthest from the door having come off the worst; and this was the place that we should have been in had the sergeant not happened to find a 'better 'ole'.

In the morning I met the Major. 'Not looking too good this morning, Doc.,' he said, scrutinising me. 'Just a moment, sir,' I replied, and took him to the shelter. He stood for some seconds silently regarding the bodies, then, having gravely saluted the dead, he turned to me and said, 'Forget it, Doc.'

We were withdrawn shortly after and the battalions being in high favour were given the best billets in the rest of Corbie. After a period of rest, we went in again to follow closely the attack of the 46th Division on the Bellinglese canal. The battalion did a solo attack at Joncourt, kicking off at 4 p.m., of all times, and penetrating the Fonsomme line. In this scrap, I got a piece of shrapnel through my tin hat and narrowly escaped being shot by one of my own men, who let off a revolver. I also encountered sixteen Germans, all of whom threw up their hands, which was absurd, as all I had was a stick. As we withdrew, three divisions exploited the gap in the line. We had lost heavily in holding the objectives, and were all taken out to rest at Hancourt – where we lived in corrugated-iron shelters. For his part in this action, Major Murphy, commanding A Company, was awarded the DSO and the adjutant got his medal.

At Hancourt, I did some shooting, bagging some partridges, rabbits and a hare. No one knew how to cook the hare, so I sent a note over to the versatile Major Marshall, who was now commanding another battalion, asking his advice. He immediately replied, giving detailed instructions, from the skinning to the serving up.

Chapter 16

The Last Scalp

Towards the end of October we moved up to a position near Bohain, being billeted in a village named Bouvry. A few tired shells fell in, and around, the village. A poor old woman who had lived in the cellar for four years, on seeing the British, decided that she could now sleep upstairs. That very night a shell landed in her bedroom and all that remained of her could have been put in a couple of sandbags. This move occupied several days. Major Marshall having left us, and the CO being on leave, Major Murphy now commanded us. This officer had had many vicissitudes with the battalion, and on occasions I had been of some service to him.

We halted one evening in the old Hindenburg system, the mess being in a trench-mortar emplacement. On these occasions, I made myself responsible for procuring and lighting a fire for the mess. Sergeant Jeffries and I found an iron cylinder about 3 ft high by 12 ins across, with a grid in the middle, and an opening below. This, which weighed about ½ cwt, we rolled to the door of the mess. I picked it up to carry it inside. As I humped it up, I heard the adjutant tell someone to get a stretcher from the cart, for the CO. (If you want to lose your stretchers give them to officers to sleep on.) As it happened, I had saved several slightly-damaged stretchers, useless for their proper purpose, but quite good as beds. I suggested to the adjutant that one of these should be used. He replied that he was getting one from the cart. I pointed out that this was absurd when there were others at hand.

'You cannot take the CO's stretcher,' he said angrily.

I replied that if there were no others, I would be glad to get one myself from the cart for the CO. He ticked me off again and told me not to be awkward whereby, losing all patience, I hurled the heavy cylinder into the mud at his feet, and at the same time exclaiming, 'You can light your own bloody fire,' and went off to the aid post. Towards mess time I tidied up, and went round to see what kind of tune the band was playing!

The fire burned brightly, a cloth was on the table, and a bottle of champagne had appeared from somewhere. I went in, expecting at best a cold silence. Instead, I was greeted cheerily, and the adjutant himself poured me out a glass of champagne, our little argument never being mentioned. A day or so later, I was riding with the Major, when he turned in his saddle and addressed me:

'Sir!'

'Light your own ---------- fire,' he chuckled, and added. 'You know I should have put you both in clink.'

'I hope you had a good night on the stretcher, sir?'

'I never got it,' he replied, 'after that bust up, I slept on the floor.'

We relieved a battalion in the line on the Oise-Sombre canal, to the right of Landrecies, taking over in the evening. The aid post was a good house on the side of the main road. I asked the medical corporal of the outgoing unit where the front line was, and when he said 1,000 yards ahead, asked if we could not get a post farther forward, but he said that there was no shelter. I then asked where his MO was and he mentioned a village three miles farther back! When it became light we went out, and seeing some chimneys rising over the hilltop, made towards them, and entered the village of Ors. This village was held jointly by friend and foe, the Oise-Sombre canal forming the dividing line between the two forces. I found some good cellars under the Brasserie, the tall chimney of which probably accounted for its unpopularity as a billet.

C Company HQ was across the road, a little in rear of us. The village had been hurriedly evacuated by the inhabitants. There were rabbits in the hutches, fowl in the backyards, and in some cases a meal remained upon the table. The rabbits got short shrift, soon finding their way into a stew-pot, but the fowls being thin and athletic, were difficult to catch. Also, in chasing your hen down the street, you had to catch it, or head it off before it reached the church, as once you passed the corner of the building, you were in full view of the German sentry on the opposite bank of the canal, less than 100 yards away! Our tall chimney certainly seemed to attract fire, and when two gas shells burst in the yards, we were in some distress. For a time it seemed a question as to whether it was best to chance the HE outside, or choke in the cellar. However, heaps of paper lighted on the floor dispersed the worst of the fumes. There was a piano in one of the sitting rooms and this was dragged down into the cellars, which we made as comfortable as possible with other furniture from the house.

Chapter 17

A Hero's End

One afternoon, scrounging around, I found a yellow double-breasted waistcoat, an old black tail-coat, and a top hat of the old-fashioned square variety. These, with a pair of field-glasses, I donned after dark, and made my way towards Company HQ. Just in time I remembered the sentry on the road, and hastily changed my hat until I had passed him. I knocked on the door of the HQ and asked a gaping orderly if 'Mr Owdfield were at home' and, pushing past him before he recovered sufficiently to stop me, entered the mess. Blank astonishment presently gave way to roars of laughter. Everyone tried on the hat, and I was just in time to have roast chicken.

BHQ, which had been located some 2,000 yards in the rear, now moved up into the village and we got orders to attack. On the afternoon previous to the action, a corporal from one of the companies was sent to me, he having received a chit to report to the FA for dental treatment. For some reason I could not send him on that day, and strictly speaking I should have returned him to his company. Fate seemed to have taken a turn in his favour. I had not the heart to do it, and told him that he could spend the night in the post, and consider himself officially evacuated. He turned out to be an excellent pianist and we soon had him on the instrument. Captain Oldfield and some officers came in during the evening, and we had a merry time roaring all the songs of the day. Oldfield was in great form, shouting out at the end of one chorus the prophetic words, 'We're going to finish the blinking war tomorrow.' With many a cheer-i-oh they left early, to get as much sleep as possible before zero hour.

The attack commenced at 5 a.m. (4 November), three divisions, the 1st, 32nd and 66th taking part. On our immediate left were the 16th Lancashire Fusiliers, commanded by Major Marshall. The canal had to be bridged. The MR Bridge was successfully erected, largely due to the gallantry of Lieutenant Kirk, who took a machine gun over on a raft and, setting the gun up on the opposite bank, kept the enemy busy. He was repeatedly wounded, but continued the fire until he fell dead across his gun. Meanwhile, two platoons had got across. Lieutenant Kirk was awarded the VC.

The LFs were less successful and here Major Marshall's great career came to an end in a gallant attempt to get his men across. He was posthumously awarded a long-merited VC. It seemed hard luck that he should fall at this time, but he would have been bitterly disappointed at the abrupt termination of the war, and at the events which followed.

Another who went west was Captain McKenzie (MR). Old Mac, as he was affectionately called, might have been safely in England, had he taken advantage of a wound received at Vermandovillers. As to the Major, he was officially medically unfit (from wounds) before he joined us! The LFs eventually crossed by the Manchesters' bridge. When we (of the RAP) crossed, I found Major Murphy on the main street and asked him how far I could go down towards our left flank.

'As far as ------ well like,' he said.

My batman, Walter Bennett, and I, set off, and presently seeing a man lying in the middle of an orchard or paddock, and thinking that he might be alive, went over to him. He was dead enough, shot through the left eye, but we stayed sometime to collect his effects. We then punched on, on a left incline, towards a coppice. Suddenly a concealed machine gun spat forth, and twigs blew from the tress around us. We did a bunk. The Major was still on the road when we got back, chuckling heartily.

'By George, Doc.,' he said, 'I never expected to see you again.'

A tank lumbered up and went forward to deal with the machine gun. I hope that the gunner survived, for I feel he could easily have scuppered us while we were looking at the dead man. We then brought our stuff over, and established a temporary post. During this scrap one of my squad leaders, Corporal Crabbe, picked up a wounded MR near the LF aid post, and had him carried there. The MO cursed him and told him not to bring any more Manchesters here to-day. Crabbe retired in good order, and shortly afterwards, finding another wounded man near the same spot, had him carried to the LF post. Out came the MO in a great rage.

'Didn't I tell you not to bring any more cases here today?' he shouted.

'Very good, sir,' said Crabbe, 'this is a Lancashire Fusilier. What would you like us to do with him?'

I have nothing to boast about in connection with the late war, but this I will say. No Allied soldier was ever turned away from my post without attention. My bearers had orders to pick up *any* wounded man (with preference to our own regiment, other things being equal) and either to bring him to me, or to take him to his own RAP, whichever happened to be the nearest. We attended to a man's wounds first and took note of his regiment afterwards!

Next morning Sambreton (the final objective) was in our hands. I went up there and secured a post – a fair-sized room with bunks round the walls, and a stove; also a small chamber at the back for me – OK. The Maltese cart arrived, and this I seized in spite of the TO, who said that it had had a long day. It was my cart anyway, and I took it back for the stuff. We loaded up and turned right, along the road from our billet, but met a string of heavy transport. The road was narrow and the hub of a huge wagon driven by an Indian, caught the hub of our cart, knocking the cart into the ditch, and bringing the sturdy pony down in a sitting position on the edge of the road, where he looked ridiculous. I reported the Indian to a passing staff officer, who said fatuously, 'You must get your men on to the wheels of the cart.'

This was exactly what we meant to do as soon as the road was sufficiently clear. With a mighty heave, in which the RAMC squad assisted, we got the cart out, and turned left after the transport, having been told that the other road was now impassable. It may have been a better road, but it was a darned bad one, and a mighty long way round.

Once or twice, we had to heave over the fields to avoid bad places. At one point, skirting a huge shell hole, the mud was halfway up to the knee. The pony stumbled and, knocking the driver down, stepped on his face. He was up again at once, however, ready to carry on. After a short breather, we all attached ourselves to the cart, and as Pollit shouted to the horse, with much heaving and gasping, we rushed through the morass. It was dark and raining, when at long last a turn brought us on to the Sambreton road, and we pulled up at the billet. Lights and voices came from within; a good fire crackled in the stove, and – the place was full of Jocks! Our billet had been jumped. Entering, I asked them what they were doing there.

'Our billet,' they said.

''our mistake," I said, 'it's been mine for several hours.'

They protested that they had been put in there.

'Then now, you get out,' I said.

'We have an officer,' said one.

'Good then, produce him.'

The officer appeared. 'I am afraid you are in my billet, sir,' I said firmly, but civilly.

'Yes, I admit we are out of our area,' he said. 'Come on boys, we'll have to go.'

I was loathe to turn those boys out into the rain, but you have to look after your own and yourself. I was, therefore, glad to answer his enquiry by telling him that he was welcome to the loft.

Chapter 18

'La Deliverance'

The inhabitants of Sambreton had welcomed us with open arms on our first entry, carrying cups of coffee out to the road with cries of 'La Deliverance'. BHQ was a great success at a large farm, the good lady regaling us with red wine that had been hidden since 1914. The old lady in our billet had broken the frame of her spectacles, and these we repaired to her great delight. She grumbled that she had no one to fetch her potatoes for her. There was living in the house a girl, about twenty years of age, and we indicated her as a likely messenger. The old lady at once broke into voluble French. But certainly not! Rather she would starve! God forbid that the girl would touch her precious potatoes. We were at a loss to understand this outburst, until the old lady suddenly cried out, 'Sale femme, coucher avec le Bosche!'

On the day after our effort with the cart, Captain Taylor led me to a stable, where I saw nineteen wounded Germans. They had been abandoned so hurriedly that they all had on hospital labels. They expected nothing short of death, and were amazed when they were fed, and more so when they found that we meant to treat them as human beings. One had his shoulder heavily bandaged and indicated by guttural grunts that it was giving much pain. Taking off the dressing I found a long vertical wound at the back of the shoulder. There was also a large bruise on the front of the upper arm, the skin in the centre of which was just beginning to break. There was marked irregularity to be felt on the front of the arm, but on further examination I concluded that the bone was not broken.

Taking a pair of scissors I slit the skin over the bruise and probed with a pair of artery forceps. The forceps struck something solid and I closed them on the object, locked them, and lifted. The other Germans were watching intently and gave vent to a chorus of 'Achs' and 'Oughs',

92

as I drew forth a complete 18-pounder nose-cap! It could only have entered by the wound at the back of the shoulder, and how it had come to rest in its final position without either fracturing any bones or tearing any vital structures in the axilla will always be a mystery to me. I got the prisoners away to hospital next day, but in the meantime two of them died.

I had considerable practice amongst the civilians also. Many children had terrible scabby and verminous heads, and we did a good amount of barbering, first, however, having to assure the French mothers their daughters would not become blind as a result of having their hair cut. One old man, wounded in the arm, said to me, 'Anglais obu tombre, Quatre Bosche, cinq cheval, tue, moi blesse, Bon!'

On an evening soon after arrival at Sambreton, I dropped in on one of the companies. On the mess were the adjutant, a company officer or two, and a very harassed-looking sergeant. (CSM, I think) whom I will call Grey. It appeared that on the night of the action, this sergeant had reached a certain barn, and had remained there for the night, re-joining his company in the morning. The adjutant was now accusing him of neglect of duty in not finding his company the night before. The sergeant, in his defence, maintained that apart from him being dead beat and lost, the adjutant had told him to stay where he was. This the adjutant denied, and continued to tell the sergeant off, reminding him that he was a warrant officer, and as such had great responsibilities. He advised Grey to accept a regimental punishment. This the sergeant stoutly refused, demanding a court martial, and further discussion followed. It was, of course, no affair of mine, but sitting there in a corner and listening to all that was said, it seemed to me that the sergeant's words rang true.

In the morning my bearer Crabbe reported sick. As he had temperature of over 102, I proposed to send him to hospital. He asked me not to do so. I pointed out to him that there was every possibility of our moving forward at any time, and that he would be running a considerable risk, but he still begged to be allowed to remain with the battalion. After some further conversation, he confided to me the real reason for wishing to stay. He had been in the barn with Grey on the night in question, and lying in the shadow of the wall, had not only seen the adjutant enter, but had heard and memorised everything that he had said. Enough! I told him that he could stay, but that he must not leave the aid post. Yes, he could communicate with his company. I gave him treatment, and had a shakedown made for him in my room.

In the evening, I found the adjutant alone in the mess. In the course of conversation, I brought up the matter of Sergeant Grey. The adjutant was reticent on the subject.

'Well,' I said, 'if I were you I would not press the charge too far. There is a martial witness in Grey's favour.'

He mumbled something about the unlikelihood of the witness being forthcoming.

'He will be forthcoming,' I said, 'for he is in my charge – sick and excused duty.'

'Then it is your duty to send him to hospital.'

'At my discretion,' I said.

He blustered about the imminence of a move, and as good as ordered me to send Crabbe to hospital, at which, without using the actual words, I gave him to understand that I would see him in hell first! What the actual upshot of it all was I never knew. The adjutant was not likely to tell me, and discipline forbade that any 'other ranks' should do so, but shortly afterwards Grey had the honour of being sent home with the Colour Party, and thereafter, whenever he saw me, he accorded me the smartest of salutes. Major Murphy got a Bar to his DSO for his command of the battalion during this action, and the adjutant got a second decoration.

We were formed up on the road ready to go forward and waiting only for the LFs to clear the crossroads. There was a commotion at the head of the column, and the adjutant galloped down the line, speaking to company commanders. The OC rear-guard tuned to us, 'Party 'shun! The War will be over in ten minutes! Stand at ease! Stand at ease! Easy!'

So, it was all over at last.

Chapter 19

Occupation of the Rhineland

The Armistice made no difference to our move. At the end of a day's march, we billeted ourselves in a village, moved on again next day and, arriving in Avenes, occupied quarters said to have been vacated by Ludendorff. Shortly after this I went on leave, in which I considered myself fortunate as rumours had it that we were to march into Germany through the forest of the Ardennes and comforting tales were told about the bitter cold in that region and the packs of wolves which would undoubtedly account for some of us.

On return from leave I found that the battalion were in Rance (Belgium), some eighty kilometres beyond the railhead and, making my way there by road, arrived just in time to play rugger against the Artillery. It was not far to the ground, but we went in state in a GS wagon drawn by four horses and with a flag flying. We beat the Artillery 15-0, and each time we scored enthusiastic supports sent up rockets and Verey lights. From there we did a two days' march to a place called Assesse in Belgium, spending the night at Yvoir in the valley of the Meuse, a delightful spot, which must have been very beautiful in the summer. Not so Assesse, where we spent several weeks. It was a gloomy village and during our stay there, whenever it failed to snow, rain fell. The earth privies in the place were all overflowing, and the Belgians had developed a habit of going round the corner of the house for sanitary purposes. We spoke to the Burgomaster about this and asked him to remonstrate with the inhabitants.

'But certainly,' he said, 'I will call the attention of the people to the matter – on Sunday in Church!'

We played Rugger, soccer and hockey, in all of which I joined until a blow from a hockey ball broke my jaw. Our Rugger team would have been a good one, but demob had started and we were constantly losing players.

The battalion left Assesse to march to Namur on a frosty morning early in February, the roads being coated with hard slippery snow and ice. The Maltese cart was loaded up with all sorts of stuff, including a sack of potatoes given to my orderlies by the friendly Belgians, so that we had difficulty in getting it up the hills, but at length we entered the town with the men roaring the chorus of 'Yack-i-hac-i-doolah'.

We entrained for Germany at 1 a.m. The train was dilapidated, with many broken windows, the night was perishing cold, and all we had in the way of food during our twelve-hour journey was some kind of soup at a wayside station. Our destination was Bonn, but we detrained at Buel, on the south bank of the Rhine, where we arrived about 1.30 p.m. The battalion crossed the bridge in artillery formation, with fixed bayonets, preceded by the band. A biting wind was blowing and, shivering with cold and hunger, I fell in behind the first company. The German population stood about on the pavements looking surly and furtive, but there was no disturbance.

We marched right across the town and were billeted in the Rhinedorf Barracks, the officers occupying NCOs' quarters (German officers always slept in private houses). The Rhinelanders soon became friendly enough. They were relieved not to have the French in occupation, and also the Canadians, for that matter, who had taken everything that they wanted at the point of a revolver and had told them that the English would be much more fierce and dominating. Soon the children were following the band, which played the new guard up to the bridge daily.

This guard was mounted and changed with the most rigid ceremonial. Bonn was a fine clean town, and German civilisation certainly appeared to be ahead of ours in some respects. A wide cinder-track ran beside the Rhine for two miles or more, and along this we used to gallop madly, scattering the strollers and giving them one more proof of the oddity of the English, since their own officers never rode at any pace other than a stately walk.

Chapter 20

Buel and Bonn

It soon became noticeable that the inhabitants of Buel invariably doffed their hats when they saw us, while those of Bonn took no notice. The explanation was that a British officer had one day had trouble with his horse in Buel, and the people had jeered him. They were given the choice of either paying a heavy fine or taking off their hats whenever they saw a British officer. They decided to take off their hats. This rather pleased the people of Bonn, as there was no love lost between the two places. Where the great bridge connecting the two towns was built, the people of Buel refused to contribute to the cost, and so the architect carved on the buttress at the Buel end the figure of a boy with his buttocks pointing towards Buel as a sign, it is said, of the contempt of the burghers of Bonn for those of Buel.

Meat was, of course, strictly rationed and the Germans were under a curfew order. One night a sentry saw two shadows emerging from an entry apparently carrying something heavy. He challenged and got no answer. He then clicked home the bolt of his rifle. At this the men dropped their burden and fled. The sentry found a large freshly-killed pig, and the brigadier was so pleased with the vigilance of the sentry that he presented the carcase to the company, who made a whoopee! Most Germans had not tasted flesh for many a day, and of soap and chocolate they had none. A bar of chocolate was sufficient to win the favour of any fraulein, and for a small cake of soap a German woman would wash all your clothes free of charge, keeping the balance of the soap for her own laundry.

When a battalion entered new quarters, a German would quickly appear and bid for the slops to feed his animals. Fraternisation was forbidden and there were strict orders against giving anything away to the enemy. Whilst there, a man appeared before the military court charged with giving away a cartload of horse manure to the people with whom he was billeted. Asked how he came to get himself into trouble by this foolish act, he said, 'Well, sir, I'm courting the daughter and I thought I ought to show them some consideration.'

What we had often heard about the attitude of the Germans to their womenfolk seemed to be borne out by observation. Not only would a German stalk ahead of his wife, but men boarding a public vehicle would push their way in without any consideration for the women in the crowd, and it appeared never to occur to a German to give up his seat to a lady. At first, we used to give up our seats to German women, but this did not always work out as expected. A colonial – New Zealand, I think – one day rose to give his seat to a female, when a male German promptly took it! This was too much for the New Zealander, who promptly seized the German by the ear and jerked him to his feet. This attitude received official sanction from a brigadier, who noticing a British officer rise to give his place to a German woman said. 'Don't do that. Make the Germans get up. Only when all male Germans are standing, give your seat to a lady.'

Thereafter it became the custom to nudge the nearest German, and say, 'Sitzplatz fur damen.'

Up to the date of ratification of peace terms, we rode free on all trams and trains. Tram fare was 25 pfennigs for any distance. All money was paper, and 25pf. (worth about a farthing) was represented by a piece of paper like a dirty tram ticket. We used to throw this small change away or give it to the nearest urchin, but after 28 June 1919, it became useful for fares. You could buy from the trams a *knipscarten,* a large ticket divided into six spaces, which was sold for the price of five tickets, a hole being punched in one of the spaces for each journey. The trams were all single-deckers and consisted of two coaches, the driver being well protected in a closed-in cabin, though there appeared to be no objection to joining the driver in his cabin if the tram was crowded. A four-coach tram started from near the bridge and, passing through Buel, became an electric railway running out into the country for fifteen or twenty miles. At the stations were level crossings, and as the train approached two large poles descended cutting off the road traffic.

The German mark soared, and when we drew on the field cashier, we received a huge wad of fifty-mark notes. The military rate differed from the civil rate, and some enterprising people did profitable financial juggling by means of postal orders from home. We knew of a change of rate before the civilians and, having drawn at the new rate, could hastily buy at the old satisfaction. The Germans were compelled to sell any article at the price marked in the window if one so demanded.

As brigade Rugby representative I was called on one day to supply two players at very short notice. I decided to play myself, and sending for my batman, W. Bennett, detailed him to play.

'Rugby, sir?' said Bennett, in some perplexity, for though a competent soccer player, his knowledge of Rugby was mainly theoretical. However, faithful unto death, and doubtless murmuring his favourite word, 'optimistic,' he donned his 'fighting kit'. As we approached the field, I instructed him that it was his duty to bring any opponent seen carrying the ball to earth, by a process of lowering his own head and seizing his enemy by the legs. In the course of the game a huge forward wearing a Harlequin jersey hurtled down the field. Directly in his path stood Bennett, who was a midget by comparison. Mindful of his orders, Bennett 'went low' and received the Harlequin's knee full in the face but, clinging on in desperation, brought down his foe.

'Eh, sir,' he said, raising a swollen face after the game, 'but did you see me fell Goliath?'

Now when the Armistice had been signed, I thought innocently that I would go home, and applied for demob. A formidable document had to be filled up and, as I was unable to state that I had any particular job to go to, the application was refused. At the same time it was pointed out to me that the contract that I had signed in 1917 was not, as I imagined 'For the duration of the War,' but 'Until the termination of the present emergency,' and, as we were still officially at war with Turkey, the emergency still existed.

When we had been in Germany for some weeks, I, with others, was asked to give a verbal undertaking to serve on the Rhine for twelve months. If you said 'Yes' it meant a substantial rise in pay; if 'no' you would probably be retained just the same at the old rate of pay. I gave the undertaking, and a couple of weeks later learned to my disgust that the 2nd Manchester Regiment was to be sent home to refit for service in India. The veterans of the war were to be relieved by battalions of young soldiers – lads who were too young to be sent out in 1918. There came a morning when I woke to the sound of shots and shuffling of feet in the barrack square, and then Bennett, bringing in my tea, announced that the Young Soldiers' Battalion had arrived. Looking out of the window while dressing, I saw these lads standing hunched up in groups round their piled arms, and my heart went out to them as I remembered our own frozen and foodless journey. Sympathy was wasted, however. They had travelled in comfort and had been fed to repletion!

Later in the morning, the 2nd MR paraded for the last time as a Great War unit and, after inspection by the brigadier, the divisional general and Lord Plumer, marched out to new quarters. I fell in behind them for the last time, and this was the only occasion on which I saw their colours unfurled. About a hundred and fifty of our temporary men, who were not yet eligible for demob, were drafted to the 51st Young Soldiers Battalion along with two or three officers, so I at once went to the ADMS and asked to be transferred to the 51st Young Soldiers in order to be with my friends.

The 2nd MR did not leave immediately, however, and before they left a rugger match was arranged – the Remnants of the 2nd MR *versus* the 51st YS. We had not full sides – I think that the Remnants had twelve men. The Remnants won 12-6, the aid post party being prominent in this engagement. Bennett scored the first try. Crabbe (now AP Corporal) the second, and a stretcher-bearer the third, while I got the last myself. I begged to be allowed to travel to England with the cadre of the 2nd MR and return at once, but this was not allowed, so I did the next best thing, by rising at 4 a.m. to see the last of the battalion I loved so well. A great lot of lads!

Two years ago I saw the present battalion give a very smart performance in a tattoo, and later visited the camp. Not being able to find the battalion, I enquired for the Manchester lines, and was told that I was in them. Alas! The old dog-fight that we used to wear on our tin hats were no more but had been replaced by a cap-badge in the shape of a grenade.

The Young Soldiers Battalion (51st YSB) was a vastly different unit from the 2nd MR. They were officered by men who had been invalided at home from active service and as each officer wore the uniform and badges of the old unit; the effect on parade was somewhat odd. Some had Glengarries instead of khaki hats, and one officer in the battalion wore a kilt! The old battalion practically ran itself, but these men still required spoon feeding to a large extent. The number that turned up on my first sick parade did not please me, and to my disgust I found half a dozen cases of scabies amongst them – more than I had seen in months of the old battalion, where, by a process of regular inspection, we had practically eliminated the disease. In fact, it was not only the 51st Battalion but all the new battalions were riddled with the disease, a sad reflection on medical supervision in England. I kept the parade together and, standing on the steps of the aid post, gave them an educational address. The Colonel was a good-natured, easygoing fellow, and he and Murphy certainly got on well together.

Before many weeks had passed, we were ordered to take over the outpost line some miles beyond Bonn. We proceeded in leisurely fashion, resting for some days in a village *en route*. Here, the QM, myself, and two other officers had a little mess on our own. There were fowls in the yard, so we asked the housewife for some fresh eggs. She shook her head, raised her hands to heaven and declared in German that she had none. We pointed to the hens, but she continued to make negative signs. 'Wait,' said the QM, and disappeared for a few minutes. He returned with a small portion of dripping in the palm of his hand, which he held under the lady's nose. She at once opened a drawer full of eggs, and thereafter we had as many as we wished, plus the run of the Frau's store of preserved vegetables and fruits!

On the outpost line, each company had its own village, with BHQ at a place called Birlinghoven. The countryside was intensely cultivated with no hedges between the fields, and very little pastureland. Though they were ahead of us on towns, in the country the Germans appeared to be more primitive than our own farming class. For instance, cows turned out to pasture had a youth squatting beside them, to keep them on their proper ground while they grazed their fill. Cattle were largely used for the traction of carts and barrows, pulling by the head, a leather band passing across the forehead below the horns. Every small bit of pasture belonged to someone. On a narrow grass verge by the roadside, you would see a solitary cow with its inevitable small attendant. The industry of the German peasants was great. Before one crop was properly off the ground, preparations would be begun for another. While the cut corn was still drying, the plough would be at work between the rows of stalks.

Living amongst these placid and seemingly friendly people, we were amused when we heard that a movement was afoot to murder us all and treated this as latrine humour. However, one morning we were all summoned to the orderly room where the Colonel read out to us a document, stating that it was known that the Workers and Soldiers Council in the unoccupied areas had decided that all British and French officers should be murdered on a certain date, and that the plot was organised so that all the murders should take place simultaneously. We were ordered to wear loaded revolvers at all times except when playing football; no one was to go out alone after sunset; and no officer was to sleep alone in his billet – as some officers were billeted in somewhat isolated farmhouses. At the same time the Burgomasters of all towns and villages were written to, told that the plot was known to British authority and advised that if a single British or French officer was murdered in the area under their jurisdiction, they would be shot without trial.

In our quiet village it was hard to realise the necessity of these precautions, and I felt rather foolish when wandering round a small brick factory with a loaded revolver in holster, amongst workmen intent only on their daily task. I slept over the aid post and on the first night placed my revolver on the locker by my bed. Then I looked at the door, which was rather a rickety affair. It seemed rather craven to lock it, but I realised that if anyone did come in quietly with a bayonet I should get the benefit of it before being able to reach the revolver. I therefore locked the door at bedtime, opening it again as a soon as I woke after daylight.

One evening a report came from Steildorf that a man was injured. I jumped on to a signaller's bicycle, and pedalled off, and had got about halfway along the lonely road before I remembered the order about not going out alone after dark. I found a man with a badly injured back – a gunner, who had no business to be in that village! The gunners had been billeted there at one time and had made friends with some of the female sex – fraternisation or no fraternisation. On this night three of them had borrowed horses from the lines and ridden over to see their girls. Realising that they had stayed too long, and being somewhat full of ale, they made a dash for their horses. My patient, on attempting to vault on his horse, had gone right over the beast. Naturally, he was much averse to going to hospital but, as he was quite helpless, I had to send for the ambulance.

The date fixed for our 'execution' passed and the plot was soon forgotten. The weather was glorious, our rations were plentiful, and life was very pleasant in our country retreat but, as I said once before, all this was too good to last. We got a new Colonel!

Chapter 21

'Corkey'

The new CO was a regular soldier, who had served in two campaigns, and his arrival was as the effect of a huge stone cast into the placid pool of our existence. The Young Soldiers required discipline and needed to be brought up to a good standard of efficiency in view of the possible necessity of an advance, but he went too far in his gingering up and, lacking discrimination, time after time he sent a man up for court martial. The brigadiers would return the case as one not requiring such procedure. The old hands particularly resented this attitude. It was all very well in the early days of the war. Then, you expected to be hustled and kicked into shape, but after having come through the campaign, men did not expect to be chivvied like raw recruits. In a short time he had so alienated his officers that they would only do just what they were told, and my own relations with him were but little better. One day I was leaning over a table in the mess reading the paper, when I heard a footstep behind me, and someone said 'good morning'. Thinking that it was one of my friends, I replied simply, not moving until an explosion occurred in the rear. I straightened up at once and apologised, but he held it against me. He had bursts of benevolence, and sometimes when meeting a man on the road would say, 'You don't look very well, my lad. You had better go and see the doctor.' Then, having sent several men in this way, he would complain about the size of the sick parade! Also, he would poke his nose too much into the personal duties of his junior officers – a thing that no good CO should do.

There came a day when he decided to have medical inspection of the whole battalion by companies and ordered me to meet him on the road in Birlinghoven. I was there with my horse in good time. The hour passed and he had not arrived. I gave him a few more minutes, and then, knowing that the first company would be waiting for me, and that the men were in all probability stripped in readiness, I mounted the Nobbler and galloped the two miles to Steildorf.

Arriving there I hurried inspection, to make up for time lost, and mounting again cantered over the field to Bucharroff. Corkey, who had started sometime after me, arrived at Steildorf just in time to see the tail of my horse disappearing over the hill towards Bucharroff. He made his own inspection, and rode after me, arriving again in time to see Nobbler's hindquarters rounding the bend for Ramsheid. The Nobbler could gallop some, and loved it, and had this kind of steeplechase gone on all day the CO would never have caught me. As it was, I approached Birlinghven again from another direction without having seen him. He was naturally much annoyed, but under the circumstances could say nothing.

The battalion had to be prepared to move forward if peace terms were not ratified on 28 June. With this in view, I asked for stretcher-bearers from each company for training. Only one company sent me. I reported this to the adjutant but got no reply. I complained again, at the same time drawing attention to the fact that my water and sanitary personnel were not up to strength, but nothing was done. I proceeded then to train those men who had been sent to me. The CO suggested that I was rude to him, but he was not above reproach himself in this respect.

The Sanitary Corporal had been demobbed, and for some time a man named Scanlon had been doing the duty very efficiently. I sent a chit into the orderly room recommending that this man be made 'sanitary corporal'. The chit was returned to me crumpled up in the hand of a private soldier – not even in any envelope – and by way of reply the one word 'No' was scrawled in red pencil across my writing! Just why I kept this document I don't know, but it was of value later and, had I retained other concrete evidence, things might have gone hard with Corkey.

Matters reached a climax at the end of June. We were to move to the neighbouring village of Dambroich, to be ready to plunge forward from there, if all did not go well on the 28th. The reason for this little move was apparent only to the Brass Hats. On the day before the move, the CO assembled all the officers in a small house, and questioned everyone as to their preparedness. He got more or less satisfactory answers from his company commanders. My turn came!

'Your people are all right, doctor?'

'No, sir,' I said briefly, and in answer to his expostulation told him of my deficiencies. Why had I not told him?

I replied that I had informed the adjutant, which I believe to be the correct procedure. In fairness to the CO, I must admit that this adjutant was not a particularly capable person and would have done better as an NCO. The conference broke up to an atmosphere of gloom, most officers leaving with a flea in their ear.

In the morning we moved at an early hour. From the first corner of the road the roofs of Dambroich could be seen less than a quarter of a mile away, but there was more fuss and flurry over the tiny move than there would have been had the old battalion been ordered to move a hundred miles at an hour's notice. Corkey certainly got a move on, and my full complement of stretcher-bearers, water, and sanitary personnel, were at once despatched to me, arriving most unhappily at the hour of sick parade and standing outside that hut along with the sick men to wait my inspection. The hut stood at the back of an open space facing the road, and presently the brigadier and his staff rode into the village.

'Who are these men?' asked the brigadier of one of his immaculate satellites. The officer made enquiry and reported, 'The sick parade, sir.'

The brigadier looked again, and nearly had a fit, for he saw what he took to be a sick parade some sixty strong. Chewing his moustache, he urged his horse forward, and must have at once got on to Corkey, for a few minutes later, Major D., a somewhat obtuse person, and without any reference to Colonel's compliments – for Corkey sent compliments to none – said, 'The Colonel wants to know if you can't get the number of this sick parade down a bit?'

I had now reached a stage of resentment that knew no discretion, and rising behind the table, I replied, 'Yes I could, and I would, if the Colonel would give me a free hand, but it is my opinion that the Colonel encourages the men to go sick.'

Major D. stared at me for a moment and left the hut. An hour or two later I was coming down the road from the mess when I met the CO. He ran at me open-mouthed. 'What do you mean by going behind my back and saying that I don't back you up?'

'I don't consider that you do, sir,' I replied, standing stiffly before him.

He then commenced a tirade, accusing me of every sort of neglect of duty, including amongst other things that, on the day of the 'steeplechase',

I had never inspected any companies at all. To all this I replied with more vigour than discretion, until at length he said, 'Well, put it on paper, for I mean to take the matter to higher authority.'

'Very good, sir,' I said, saluting him smartly as he turned away.

I put it on paper, to the extent of two pages of foolscap, finding some satisfaction in telling Corkey just what was in my mind, and concluding my effort with the statement that I had had the honour to serve with the 2nd MR under five different COs with all of whom I had been in perfect accord.

A day or two later I was riding back over the fields to Burlinghoven when I met three officers. They grinned widely as I approached, and called out, 'Cheer–i-oh, Doc. We've heard about you,' delighted that at last someone had answered back. I was a popular hero, but also was in the soup, and dearly wished that Colonel Sampson, our old ambulance CO was with the division to back me up. Sampson, however, had returned to England for other duty, and his successor I had never seen. In the days that followed, Corkey, of course, ignored me, but each morning, afternoon, and evening I was careful to give him the usual salutation to which he was obliged to reply.

In due course I was ordered to appear at the field ambulance and report to Colonel O'G. and set forth feeling somewhat despondent. The man knew nothing of me, and would, I felt, think the whole affair a damned nuisance. I reckoned without a loyal Irishman! At the FA I was directed to a cricket field where I found O'G., and another officer, sprawling on the grass watching the match. I reported myself to him formally.

'Ah,' he said, looking up,'"You're Parker, are you? Sit down. What have you been doing to your Colonel?"

Sitting on the grass I gave him a faithful account of all my relations with Corkey from A to Z. Meanwhile his eye travelled over me, and came to rest on my left sleeve, which bore four chevrons. One red and three blue.

'Hum,' he said, 'have you any evidence?'

I produced the chit with 'no' scrawled across it and described the manner in which it reached me.

'Ah, that's bad, or rather good,' said O'G., 'but have you any more?'

'No, I never thought that matters would come to this pass and destroyed much that might have been useful.'

'Pity! Well. You've got to appear before General YZ and I shall come with you.'

On the appointed day I called for O'G. and together we climbed to the Schloss in the forest. O'G. chatted gravely on the way up. He had evidently left no stone unturned in his investigations and was ready for battle. We entered the great hall and sat near one end. Presently Corkey arrived and stood talking to a staff officer at the other extreme of the hall, the whole atmosphere being rather suggestive of 'pistols for two'. An officer approached and informed us that the general would see us in the Round Room. This we reached by turrets and narrow corridors in the walls. The general was seated at a table in the centre of the room. Corkey sat against the wall on his right, O'G. and I on his left.

Invited to state his case, Corkey spoke in a droning voice, mentioned my rudeness to the 'Good morning' incident and stressing he had got on with one Jackson, my deputy when on leave. The general then took my statement, and read every word of it aloud, after which he invited me to defend myself. I did not say much, for indeed there was little to say that was not contained in my statement. The 'chit' was produced and condemned by the general. He was most fair, and agreed that my complaint to the adjutant was the correct and soldierly thing to do – in preference to a direct approach to the CO. The O'G. got onto his feet, and broke into an impassioned address, which caused me no little embarrassment. Never, had it appeared, had there been such a paragon of all military virtue. None so conscientious and efficient! I listened in amazement until I remembered that there was an MO still with the ambulance who had been with us during the last twelve months of the war. He, it seemed, must have given no bad account of me to O'G.

The general listened gravely while Corkey fidgeted in his chair. I had opportunity to speak further, but by this time I had begun to be curiously sorry for Corkey. He seemed a very lone figure, and if he was worsted in this case he would probably lose his command, which would be a very serious thing for him as a regular soldier. Whereas for my part, the verdict meant little. The general ruminated awhile, and then summed up the case. Here, he said, we had two officers, each actuated by the best motives, each anxious to do their duty, but who could not get on together. The obvious solution was to separate them, and to this end he suggested that I should exchange units with Jackson, the MO of the 52nd Battalion.

O'G. at once sprang to his feet. With respect he could not accept such a decision. It would be a calamity for me – would follow me into civil life and ruin me for ever, etc., etc.

He surely should have been a KC! The general listened to all, but remained unmoved, and we left the Schloss beaten on points. Corkey remained with the general.

Outside O'G. became concerned. Had he backed me up properly? Was there anything else that he should have said? I assured him that he could not have done more had he been my foster-brother. 'A pity,' he said, 'that you had not more documentary evidence, but mind you (brightening), that CO of yours isn't getting off scot free. I know YZ, and I can tell you that colonel's getting his tail twisted right now.' That evening I saw Jackson and told him of the proposed exchange. 'I shan't come,' he said briefly. 'I had enough of it while you were on leave.'

Next morning I did sick parade for the last time, and then watched my servant getting my kit together. I had had no particular regret at the thought of leaving Corkey's mob, as young Kent (late of the 2nd MR) irreverently called them, but now, on looking round at the familiar faces of my orderlies, I realised that I had several old friends, and a number of new ones, in the battalion, and that I had no wish to break fresh ground at this stage of my service. I sat down and wrote a chit requesting an interview with the CO. Reply came immediately, properly sealed in an envelope. 'Certainly, I am in the orderly room.'

I presented myself at once, being careful to observe all the formalities. The CO was alone. He sat with his forearms on the table and regarded me gloomily.

'Well,' he said gruffly.

'I thought, sir, that you might be open to a sporting offer.'

'What is it?'

'If you admit that I have tried to do my duty and if you will take back what you said to me in the road, I will volunteer to stay with you.'

'But are we going to pull together?'

'I see no reason why we should not, sir.'

Quite suddenly he half rose and stretched out his hand, and I can only hope that from that day forward I kept my part of the bargain as loyally as he did.

Chapter 22

Sentence of Death

One of the most unpleasant duties that an MO had occasionally to perform during the war was to express an opinion as to the sanity or otherwise of a man who had deserted his post in the line, well knowing that a man's life probably hung upon this decision. Duty must be done, however, and an honest opinion had to be given.

We were out at rest sometime during the summer of 1918, when a lad named Cousins was brought to me for this purpose. Actually, he could scarcely be said to have deserted, for he had wandered to a more dangerous spot, and had remained there until found sitting under a bush. It appeared that he had had bad news from home, his father having committed suicide. I had a considerable conversation with Cousins, decided that he was sane, and signed a paper to that effect. A request then came that I should give an opinion as to his mental condition ten days previously. On this point I refused to express any opinion as I had not seen him on that date mentioned. Cousins was tried and sentenced to death, but the sentence was reduced to a term of imprisonment, to be served forthwith.

At the Armistice there was a sort of general amnesty, and Cousins re-joined us at Assesse with two years suspended sentence hanging over his head. At this time opportunity was given to men physically fit to join the regulars. Cousins presented himself for examination, saying that he wished to join the regulars to redeem his character. I found him fit. Hardly had the cadre of the 2nd MR marched out of the Rhinedorf Barracks, when Cousins, who with others had been transferred to the 51st, turned up at the aid post and applied to be taken on as my batman. He was a smart clean lad, had had previous experience as an officer's servant, and I was glad to get hold of one of the old battalion. He made an excellent servant.

When we had out little mess of four, on our way to the outpost line, he bundled the other three servants into the back premises and took entire charge of the mess himself. Also, he kept us in order. We would be sitting around the fire at midday when he would appear in the room, and standing stiffly behind the head of the table, would say, 'Sit for lunch, please,' in a manner that seemed to forbid delay.

As the summer of 1919 wore on, numbers of our older men became due for demobilisation, and I had to examine each small draft for freedom from lice and scabies before they were allowed to proceed to England. One morning, I had just finished examining a small party when Cousins appeared before me.

'What is it, Cousins?' I asked, in surprise.

'For examination, sir.'

'Ah, of course, you are going home to begin your regular training?'

'No, sir, it's my ticket – demob!'

Our eyes met, and he flushed scarlet from his khaki collar to the roots of his hair. I knew that he was clean, but I put him through the routine examination, and then returning to the table, slowly picked up the pencil. The words 'Two years suspended sentence' were clearly before my mind. After all, the war was over, and my duty began and ended with ascertaining his freedom, or otherwise, from scabies and lice, if this particular orderly room could not – I signed the chit. Cousins picked up his pack, and I stood chatting with him in the doorway for a few minutes enquiring about his plans and wishing him luck. Then with a final smart salute he turned to join the little party in the road. A few days later I encountered the adjutant.

'I say, doctor,' he cried, 'that batman of yours – that fellow – your batman!'

'Yes?'

'He's gone – demobbed!'

'Yes, I was sorry to lose a good servant.'

'But – he – he was under suspended sentence.'

'Oh,' I said, opening my eyes a little wider.

'Got right away,' he continued in agitation. 'No means of tracing – no clue.'

'Well,' I said, 'All our men in the 2nd Battalion came from Lancashire; that should give you a clue.' (I knew very well that Cousins had gone to Windsor!)

As I write these lines I have before me the photograph of a smart young soldier – signed: 'Yours Obedient J. Cousins.'

With autumn came the fruit season. Most of the roads were lined with pear, plum or other fruit-bearing trees. The crops were marketed for the relief of rates, and the Germans no more thought of taking fruit then they would of cutting their neighbour's corn. It was very pleasant on a hot day to snatch a ripe plum as one rode under the tree.

Autumn wore on, and 'hurrah for rugger weather,' said Lieutenant Thwaites. Since the burial of the hatchet all had been well between the CO and myself, and with the help of Thwaites, I began to organise a battalion Rugby team, it seemed that I could do no wrong. Our entry for the Corps Championships caused some amusement since we could only muster some half-dozen active Rugby Union players. There were, however, in the ranks a number of men who had played Northern Union or, as it is now called, Rugby League, and we got one or two enthusiastic recruits from the soccer players. The CO gave every assistance and allowed me to have the men whenever I wanted them for practice or instruction. Playing seven officers and eight other ranks, we scrambled through the early rounds. Then a fly appeared in the ointment. A sergeant, who fancied himself at the game, was spreading dissension by proclaiming that there were too many officers in the team. There was only one way of dealing with this – the officers must play the rest of the battalion. I approached the CO who not only gave his approval, but though the wrong side of forty, at once consented to turn out. Including the colonel we had nine men and made up our XV by co-opting six enthusiastic novices whom we instructed in scrum formation in the ante-room after mess.

We beat the rest of the battalion 12-0, the CO himself getting a try from a line out, and criticism was silenced. To cut a long story short, we scraped through to the final, in which we met the Corps Troops who played fourteen officers (and a corporal who was no dud). The match was played on the Hofgarten in Bonn before an international crowd of about 4,000. In the first half we scored early 'according to the plan,' but the CT replied. We led again in the second half, but a few minutes before the end the CT equalised. Extra time was ordered – five minutes each way. In the first minute we scored behind the posts. Thwaites took the kick. The ball sailed straight for the goal, and then unaccountably curved outside the left-hand post. One minute from time we still held the lead but, thirty seconds later, the CT got over in the corner and our supporters gasped with relief as the kick failed.

Three days later we replayed. We were in arrears at half-time, but in the second half training and teamwork told, and we finished up a try to the good. In the evening, by special permission, the whole team dined in the Sergeants' Mess, and during the meal, an official telegram of congratulation arrived from brigade. Afterwards we crossed over to the village hall where a sing-song was in progress, at which a number of trophies for various athletic events were to be presented. It had been sprung upon us that the team were to receive medals – a somewhat embarrassing position for Rugby Union men who are not accustomed to accepting such mementoes. As there was one medal short, I suggested to the CO that I should forgo mine.

'Nothing of the sort, doctor,' he said, with a touch of his old asperity. 'You will take your medal like anyone else.'

And so, from the hands of the man with whom I had been at loggerheads, I received my only war decoration! General YZ and his staff came to dinner next night, and we duly filled them up.

I had great hopes of a match against the French Army, but before this could be arranged the Division broke up, and the 51st went home. During the summer I had signed a contract for a further six months, with the promise of certain release at the end of the period, so once more I remained behind, became unemployed and for this extraordinary reason my leave was stopped. After drifting about for a time, I was sent to the Durham Light Infantry in Cologne. Here we had a lazy life. Active service was practically over, we were billeted in the suburbs and had no effective transport.

At one end of Hohestrasse was a large German officers' club, and to this we frequently repaired in the afternoon for tea and music. A massive statue of Bismarck stood outside, and I have wondered what the old man would have thought could he have seen British officers using the club as their own. At the other extremity of the Hohestrasse there was a hotel which we called the Earwig, where one could dine and dance. Our evenings were spent in going the rounds of the cabarets. Champagne was cheap, and a round of drinks generally meant a magnum.

One of our officers had been a prisoner and he used to make a practice of hitting the first German he saw on the way home, exclaiming at the same time You made me eat grass' or 'You spat on me behind the barbed wire'. Sometimes the German would hit back, and a good scrap would follow. If home seemed too far off you could always sleep at the Earwig. Terms were strictly cash – in fact, you had to buy a food ticket before being served with a meal.

On one occasion, having put up at the Earwig, I descended in the morning to see a Durham officer sitting disconsolately at a table on which were only clean plates and cups. He brightened up on seeing me and asked if I had any money. I bought an extra breakfast ticket, and when we had settled to the meal, asked him where he had got to the night before, 'I don't really know,' he said, 'but this morning I awoke to the song of birds, and looked out on to a sea of apple trees. Then a girl came in with a cup of tea and said, "You will have to get up and go now before the neighbours wake up!" She pointed out the direction, and I walked and walked and walked, until I struck tram lines, and landed here a couple of hours ago, as hungry as a hunter. What I can tell you, he concluded, is that I had plenty of money on me last night!'

In February the Durhams went home, and for the third time I became the sole survivor. Battalions of the new Regular Army were now being sent out, to replace all the troops on the Rhine. Amidst the confusion I was posted to a battalion which I found did not exist!

My service was now fast drawing to a close, but within less than three weeks of release, I was sent over to take over the XYZs at Solingen. Taking over was now a serious business. No longer could the charmed words 'destroyed by shellfire' be used, and practically every pill had to be counted. The XYZs had served out during the war and had been home to refit. They were without exception the windiest lot I encountered. A Monarchist rising was taking place in the vicinity, and this appeared to terrify them.

Some machine-gun companies were sent up as reinforcement. These hard-bitten Western Front veterans naturally joined the battalion mess. In the war days it would have been, 'Cheer-i-oh, come in, share what we've got and good luck to you.'

Not so now! The XYZs looked down their noses at the stained and worn uniforms of the gunners and complained bitterly about the mess being overcrowded. Remarks were heard such as, 'These damned temporaries are going home while we have to say here and be murdered.'

Actually there was no danger at all. The gunners took no notice at first, but at length one of them said aloud, 'Well, I've been through the three battles of Ypres, but never in all my service have I seen so much wind up as during the last three days in this mess!'

The 23rd of March 1920 dawned and I returned to Cologne to claim my release. The officer asked me if I would like to sign a further contract. No! I would not!

'Well,' he said, 'if you won't sign we can't make you.'

'I know you can't,' I replied, and felt for once I had had the last word.

As a final stupidity he gave me an order for a train that did not run. At Boulogne red tape help me up for twenty-four hours and, having got rid of all my foreign money, I had to borrow. I arrived in London too late to report to the War Office that day, and as all hotels were full, had to sleep with a policeman who charged me ten shillings for the pleasure.

The visit to the War Office meant walking down long corridors and waiting outside doors. Once more I was asked to sign another contract, and again I declined. Now surely – but no! I must report at Caxton Hall. I arrived at this place in no good humour about 1 p.m. Could I come back at 3 p.m.? I could not! What might they want with me? It appeared that they thought I might be ill.

'There is nothing the matter with me except fair wear and tear doesn't count,' I said.

'Oh yes it does,' said the old gentleman, 'if the amount is sufficient.'

'Will it suffice if I say that I am in good health?'

'No. Pull up your shirt.'

And so the last order that I got in the army was curiously similar to the first. I adjusted my toilet. The door swung to behind me. I was free!

Conclusion

Tending the wounded, in the abstract, is a valiant occupation, but the reality is far from ideal, as shown on the battlefields of the Western Front. It is a trade with no romantic side, a business of dirt and sorrow, of danger from fire with no chance of retribution, such as the ordinary soldier has against his enemy. It is work not suddenly of heroic deeds, but of stolid endurance in the face of great and unrelenting adversity, and those who choose this path, who not necessarily built on the lines of a popular hero, have infinite capacity for suffering and endurance at the sight of torment. It is work that calls not so much for bravery as for real courage, not for spurts of endeavour, but for prolonged effort. It is defined in the sentence, 'You have to go on smiling, even when you are tired.'

After four and half years of fighting many RAMC establishments would continue in service beyond the Armistice, offering relief care in Belgium and Germany. They also continued to staff the hospitals where wounded and disabled men were being treated for continuing illnesses and impairments. With the transition from war to peace, as society slowly began to demobilise, those men who had served in the RAMC ranks now sought to pick up the threads of their civilian lives, by either returning to their old jobs or starting out on new career paths. Captain Harry G. Parker was no different, returning to Cumbria to resume his life as a medical professional. Like others, as an officer of the RAMC, he was a citizen who became a soldier for the duration of the war, returning to his civil status once it had ended.

The crucial role of the RAMC in the First World War is clearly illustrated by the substantial number of awards for gallantry that were received by all ranks. Its honour roll includes one award of the Victoria Cross, followed by a Bar, to medical doctor Noel Godfrey Chavasse and another Bar to the Victoria Cross to Arthur Martin-Leake, surgeon of the 5th Field Ambulance. In total there were 6,501 military awards including seven Victoria Crosses, 499 Distinguished Service Orders (twenty-five with Bar), 1,484 Military Crosses (184 with Bar), three Albert Medals, 395 Distinguished Conduct Medals (nineteen with Bar) and 3,002, Military Medals (199 with Bar). Like other non-combatant military units the RAMC was officially recognised in the interwar period for their service through war memorials commemorating those who died. On 13 July 1922, in the north aisle of the nave of Westminster Abbey, a fine memorial tablet was unveiled by the Duke of Connaught, Colonel in Chief of the Corps, initially paying tribute to those who died in the First World War, but today also honouring those who died in subsequent conflicts. Designed by F.J. Wilcoxson, the memorial inscription reads:

MCMXIV MCMXIX
ROYAL ARMY MEDICAL CORPS

In memory of 743 Officers and 6130 Warrant Officers, Non-Commissioned Officers and Men who fell in the Great War, and whose names are enrolled in a Golden Book placed in the Chapter House. 'They loved not their lives unto the death.'

Below on a small tablet, unveiled in 1987, is the inscription for the 1939-45 war:

And of the 437 officers and 2026 other ranks who gave their lives

The plaque was accompanied by a *Golden Book of Remembrance*, created by the novelist and calligrapher Graily Hewitt, which was initially on display in the Chapter House but now resides in a display case in front of the memorial. In 1927 a memorial window was added to the collection, comprising of two stained-glass windows designed by J. Ninian Comper. Depicting the figures of Edward the Confessor and Edwin, Abbot of Westminster, the script of the original inscription at the base read as follows: 'who gave their lives in the Great War 1914-1919.' Beneath are the names listed of those countries in which the fallen served: France, Flanders, Dardanelles, Italy, Macedonia, Mesopotamia,

Egypt, Palestine, Africa, Persia, India and Russia. This was later altered to commemorate those who died in the Second World War and now reads:

In memory of the Royal Army Medical Corps of all ranks who gave their lives in the service of their country.

In 2014 a monument, dedicated to the RAMC, was unveiled at the National Arboretum in Staffordshire. Comprising a bronze sculpture depicting a medic carrying a wounded soldier over rocky ground, it is set in a large woodland with individual trees dedicated to RAMC members. At the entrance to the wood there stands a tapering plinth complete with an inset, a brown marble tablet inscribed with the RAMC symbol, a wreath encompassing a sword with snake entwined, and name in gold.

But perhaps, the simplest tribute of all comes in the form of words:

In picturing the neat hospital ward and the sisters and orderlies at their work, trim beds and flower-decked tables, one gathers a view of only a part of the RAMC. Rather one should picture the Medical Officer who stood over the body of a wounded man on the field of action, until himself shot down, or the men of the Royal Army Medical Corps who crossed a shell-swept pontoon bridge every night to bring the wounded out from the firing line … . One should picture men sleeping in their cloaks in ploughed fields, occupying the trenches with the fighting men, wounded themselves or swept out by shell or rifle fire to things beyond humanity's ken. In all their work, 'Faithful in danger,' and, no matter what branch of service they may be called to undertake, playing a noble part.

Vivian, Charles,
With the Royal Army Medical Corps
(RAMC) at the Front

Appendix I

Timeline of Army Medical Services (RAMC sources)

1690	Regimental Surgeons already established, one commissioned per regiment/battalion
1664	Post of Surgeon General (SG) created
1673	Surgeons' Mates established in Guards and Infantry units
1685	Post of Physician General created
1686	Post of Apothecary General created
1690	Purveyors appointed to Field Officers (chosen from Staff Surgeons until 1798).
1702	First Cavalry Surgeons' Mates appointed.
1727	First Medical Officer appointed to the artillery.
1756	Post of Inspector of Regimental Infirmaries created.
1756	Army Medical Board (AMB) created. For governance of medical services. Stands down in 1763.
1793	AMB reconvened. Composes of SG, Physician General and Inspector of Regimental Infirmaries.
1793	Ordnance Medical Board founded
1804	Hospitals' Mates commissioned, initially as Hospital Assistants, then Hospital Surgeons from 1830
1808	Army Medical Department (AMD) first formed.
1810	Post of Director General (DG) created.

1853   Ordnance Medical Board merged into AMD.

1854   Hospital Conveyance Corps formed. Other ranks subsumed into Land Transport Corps.

1855   Medical Staff Corps created.

1856   AMD moves under Secretary State for War

1857   Army Hospital Corps (AHC) formed from MSC.

1870   AMD moves under the War Office

1873   Regimental surgeons move to AMD.

1873   SG re-introduced as a rank.

1873   Apothecaries cease.

1873   AMD granted authority over AHC

1879   Reserve of AMD officers granted.

1881   Officers of Orderlies become QM

1884   AHC reverts to MSC. Medical Officers of AMD grouped with QMs of the AHC.

1885   Volunteer MSC formed; includes Medical Officers as well as regular soldiers.

1888   Further AMS reserve officers formed,

1891   Hybrid rank introduced for medical officers.

1891   Militia MSC formed, includes medical officers and soldiers.

1898   ROYAL ARMY MEDICAL CORPS (RAMC) FORMED, from amalgamating the AMS with the MSC. Proper military rank now given to medical officers.

Appendix II

Battles on the Western Front in Flanders and France

Stage 1: The German Offensive – The Retreat from Mons, 23 August to 5 September 1914

- 23-24 August 1914: Battle of Mons – Initial clashes between the Germans and the Entente armies. EF begins retreat from Mons.
- 26 August 1914: Battle of le Cateau – British corps fight a holding action during the retreat.

The Advance to Aisne: 6 September-1 October 1914

- that halts the German advance into France
- 12-15 September 1914: Battle of the Aisne – The Germans retreat to ridge above Aisne. Both sides dig in.

Military Operations: The Defence of Antwerp, 4-10 October 1914. Predominantly naval troops sent to help the Belgian Army defend Antwerp.

- 10 October-2 November 1914, Battles of la Bassée, Armentieres and Messines – Whole BEF moved to Flanders from Aisne in an effort to outflank the Germans in France.
- 19 October-22 November 1914, Battle of Ypres – Often known as the First Battle of Ypres, epic fight to the east of the city which resulted in stalemate.

Stage 2: Trench Warfare 1914-1916

November 1914-February 1915: Winter operations – French orders for major offensive in December which lead to disastrous haphazard British attacks.

March to October 1915: Summer operations

- 10 March-22 April 1915: Battle of Neuve Chappelle – British Army mounts first offensive on large scale: costly in terms of casualties but results in the recapture of Neuve Chapelle.
- 22 April-25 May 1915: Battle of Ypres 1915; known as the Second Battle of Ypres, it began with a surprise German attack using poison gas.
- 9 May 1915: Battle of Aubers; catastrophic attack that cost 11,000 British casualties for no gain.
- 15-25 May: Battle of Festubert, and later Givenchy, Hooge and Bellewaarde; British called upon to continue offensive. Again, heavy cost in casualties.
- 25 September-8 October 1915: Battle of Loos – first large-scale British offensive. Also, first time the British used poison gas.

Stage 3: The Allied Offensive, 1916

24 June to 19 November: Battles of the Somme – a Franco-British offensive. Huge British losses on the first day; 15 September saw the first ever use of tanks on the battlefield.

Stage 4: The Advance to the Hindenburg Line, 1917.

Military Operations on the Ancre: 11 January – 13 March 1917 – Final flickering of the Somme offensive as British seek tactical advantage on heights above the River Ancre valley.

Military Operations: The Germans retreat to the Hindenburg Line, 14 March-5 April 1917. During the Somme fighting of 1916 the Germans constructed a formidable new defensive system some miles in the rear.

British detect the withdrawal and follow their advance, being brought to a standstill at the outer defences.

Stage 5: The Allied Offensives, 1917.

Military Operations: The Arras Offensive, 9 April-15 May 1917.

The Battle of Arras, 1917: The British were called upon once again to launch an attack in support of a larger French offensive. Opening battles, such as the Battle of Vimy, are very encouraging, but again the offensive, known as the Battle of Arras, bogs down. Attempts to outflank the German lines prove costly.

Military Operations: The Flanders Offensive, 7 June-10 November 1917.

- 7-14 June 1917: Battle of Messines: Successful offensive that resulted in the capture of the Wytschaete-Messines ridge, south of Ypres.
- 31 July-10 November 1917: Battle of Ypres, known as the Third Battle of Ypres, or more commonly Passchendaele. Enormous British casualties. Battlefield renowned for being a quagmire of mud.

Military Operations: The Cambrai Operations, 20 November-7 December 1917.

Battle of Cambrai was a British attack that employed new artillery and mass tanks. Initially successful until a German offensive stopped the advance. Ten days later, the British had regained the ground.

Stage 6: The German Offensives, 1918

Military Operations: The Offensive in Picardy, 21 March-5 April 1918:

First Battles of the Somme – German High Command commit to a series of large scale offensives. The first, Operation MICHAEL, strikes the British Fifth and Third Armies, inflicting heavy losses.

Military Operations: The Offensive in Flanders, 21 March-5 April 1918

- 9-29 April 1918, Battle of the Lys: Third German offensive with the objective of capturing key railway and supply roads and cutting off the British Second Army at Ypres. After initial success, the Germans were held back by British, Commonwealth and French Reserves.

Military Operations: The Offensive in Champagne, 1918

- 27 May-6 June: Battle of the Aisne: Small and tired British force was struck and virtually destroyed as part of another German offensive named Operation BLUCHER.

Stage 7: The Advance to Victory, 1918.

Military Operations: The Retaliation of Champagne.

- 20 July-2 August 1918: Battles of the Marne including the Battle of the Soisonnais and Qurcq (23 July-2 August) and Tardenois (20-31 July). British forces take part in successful large scale counte-offensive of the Marne.

Military Operations: The Advance in Picardy, 8 August-3 September 1918

- 8-11 August 1918: Battle of Amiens. The British Fourth Army attacks alongside French forces and scores a notable victory and a deep advance from Amiens
- 21 August-3 September 1918: Second Battles of the Somme. British Third and Fourth Armies commence offensive operation on the same ground over which the 1916 Battle of the Somme was fought. They make a deep advance.

Military Operations: The Advance in Flanders, 18 August-6 September 1918. Second and Fifth Armies begin operations in the Lys valley, recapturing the ground lost in April 1918.

Military Operations: The Breaking of the Hindenburg Line, 26 August-12 October 2018

- 26 August -3 September 2018: Second Battle of Arras. First and Third Armies attack successful from Arras and break the German Drocourt-Queant Line.
- 12 September-9 October 1918: Battles of the Hindenburg Line. A series of large-scale offensive operations that advance to and break the Hindenburg Line system. Carved out by the British First, Third and Fourth Armies.

Military Operations: The Final Advance in Flanders, 28 September-11 November 1918

- 28 September-20 October: Battle of Ypres 1918
- 14-19 October: Battle of Cambrai

The British Second Army and the Belgian Army come together to finally break out of the Ypres Salient. More ground is gained in a day than in the entire Passchendaele offensive of a year before.

Military Operations: The Final Advance in Artois, 20 October-11 November 1918.

First and Fifth Armies continue the advance in the Artois region, liberating the French coalfields, lens and Douai.

Military Operations: The Final Advance in Picardy, 17 October-11 November 1918.

The hardest fought of the final offensive actions, incorporating the Battles of the Selle, Valenciennes and Sambre. First, Third and Fourth Armies push on through the Hindenburg Line, recapturing Valenciennes and finally liberating Mons, where it had all begun for the British more than four years before.

Armistice and Advance into the Rhine
- British forces advance across Belgium, cross into Germany and take up positions on the Rhine in accordance with the terms of the Armistice of 11 November 1918.

Appendix III

Glossary of Place Names

Adinfer
A small village located approximately seven miles, (just over eleven kilometres) east of Arras. Destroyed during the war, the area still bears scars from some of the bloodiest fighting on the Western Front.

Berneville
Village located around half a mile (one kilometre) from the Doullens-Arras main road. Site of heavy fighting.

Amiens
The Battle of Amiens (8-11 August 1918) heralded the start of the Hundred Days Campaign, a four-month period of Allied success whereby the forces launched a victorious operation against the German Spring Offensive.

Le Quesnoy
Le Quesnoy was an old fortress town occupying a strategic position in north-eastern France. The Germans held le Quesnoy for almost the entire war, from August 1914 through to its dramatic liberation on 4 November 1918, when the capture of le Quesnoy, as part of the Battle of the Sambre, commenced. The battle was to consist of a series of engagements mounted by the British First, Third Fourth Armies together with the New Zealand Division across a thirty-mile (forty-six kilometre) front. Here the New Zealanders famously scaled a ladder set against the ancient walls of the town and captured any remaining German troops.

Vermandovillers	A small village in the Somme commune of northern France, approximately twenty-six miles (forty-two kilometres) east of Amiens. The Battle of Vermandovillers commenced on 24 September 1914 and the front line remained relatively stable for the next two years. The position was stoutly defended by the 11th Division of the Prussian/German Army. The village has a dedicated German War Cemetery, on the very southern end of the Somme battlefield, commemorating those who fell during the First World War. Some 22,655 men are buried here, including 13,200 buried in a *kameradengrab*, (comrades' grave) mass burial.
Château Misery	The village of Misery lies three kilometres, (around two miles) from the Somme front line and was completely destroyed during the conflict.
Cizancourt	A small village located in the Somme, in the Picardie region of northern France. All but destroyed during the war.
Peronne	Located in the district of the Somme, in the region of Hauts-du-France, northern France. Tucked into a meander of the Somme River, it is close to where all the battles of the Somme took place. The town had been the German headquarters until it was abandoned and set on fire in 1917. It was then used by the British until the German Offensive of March 1918 enabled them to regain control. Battle of Mont Saint-Quentin – in September 1918 Australian troops seized and held Mont Saint-Quentin, a hill overlooking Peronne, which was a pivotal German defensive on the line of the Somme. They finally liberated the town of Peronne a day later.

Fonsomme   The source site of the River Somme, Fonsomme lies within the commune of Aisne, in the Hauts-de-France region of northern France.

Joncourt   A small village, around six miles, (ten kilometres) north of St Quentin in Aisne, northern France. It lay immediately west of the German fortification called the Beaurevoir-Fonsomme line, often referred to as the 'Hindenburg Support Line'. The position was a series of trenches and concrete fortifications, held by the Germans. It was captured by Australian troops on 30 September 1918, finally cleared of enemy soldiers by 5th Australian and 32nd Divisions on the following day. Joncourt has two British war cemeteries, the first, East British Cemetery, is located around one kilometre east of the village and contains seventy-one First World One burials, fifty-two of which belong to the 15th or 16th Lancashire Fusiliers or the 2nd Manchesters. The Joncourt British Cemetery contains sixty-one burials, fifty-five of which belong to the 10th Argyll and Sutherland Highlanders. All graves date from the period 30 September -3 October 1918.

Bohain   Now called Bohain-en-Vermandois, the town is located in the Aisne region of Hauts-du-France, northern France. Site of the Bohain-St Quentin line during the Hundred Days offensive, 1918.

Oise-Sambre Canal   The Sambre–Oise Canal saw one of the last Allied victories in the First World War before the Armistice with Germany. Wilfred Owen, an officer and leading poet of the war, was killed as he crossed the Sambre–Oise Canal at the head of a raiding party. His friend 2nd Lt Foulkes, who was wounded in the attack, said that Owen was last seen trying to cross the canal on a raft under very heavy gunfire. Owen's death occurred only a week before the war ended, his leadership and bravery on that day gave rise to him being recommended for the Military Cross.

Landrecies

Landrecies is a small town in the Nord region of northern France, approximately twenty-five miles (forty kilometres) south-east of Valenciennes. It was the scene of rearguard fighting between British and German forces on the night of 25 August 1914. The town remained in German hands from then until it was captured by 25th Division on 4 November 1918. To the east of the town there is a communal cemetery, which was once used by the German forces to bury their own dead, but after the Armistice the German graves were removed and replaced with Commonwealth casualties. There are fifty-six burials commemorating those who fell in the First World War, including thirty graves of those who were killed during the rearguard action. Eleven burials are unidentified.

Ors

Ors is a small village located in the Nord region of northern France. It lies on the Sambre–Oise Canal, in a small wood called Bois l'Évêque. It was in the hands of the Germans for much of the First World War but was cleared by the Allied forces on 1 November 1918. It has two war cemeteries, a Communal Cemetery located at the north-west end of the village, where 63 First World War casualties are buried, four of which are identified. There is also the Ors British War Cemetery, around three kilometres north-east of the village church. Formed in November 1918, the cemetery contains 107 Commonwealth burials from this period, six of which are unidentified.

Sambreton	Village located south of Landrecies, Hauts-du-France, northern France
Rance (Belgium)	Rance is a town located in the Walloon Region of Belgium, some forty-nine miles (seventy-nine kilometres) south of Brussels.
Assesse (Belgium)	The village of Assesse is located in the Wallon province of Namur.
Albert	Albert was one of the main towns behind the lines for Allied forces. From September 1916 field ambulances and 5th Casualty Clearing Station were based here. It lies on the main road from Amiens eastwards to Bapaume, across the Somme battlefields. Albert was devastated during the war and rebuilt afterwards. The town did fall to the Germans briefly during the Somme battles but was quickly recaptured by Allied forces. There are a number of war cemeteries that lie within its environs. On the eastern outskirts is Bapaume Post Military Cemetery, which was in use from July 1916 to January 1917. Approximately 150 men were buried here during this period. Another 250 or so graves were added after the Armistice, many being men of the 34th (Tyneside) Division.

A little to the south of Albert town is the communal cemetery where there is a separate plot maintained by the CWGC. Continuing south-east from the town centre, on the same road is the Albert French National Cemetery. Here lie the graves of 3,175 French soldiers. |
| Angle Wood | Located on the Somme. Strategic position in the Battle of Guillemont. |
| Corbie | Field Ambulance. A small town situated approximately nine miles (fifteen kilometres) upriver from Amiens, it lies in the valley of the river Somme |

Old Queen's House – Isle of Wight	The secondary wing of Osbourne House, once belonging to Queen Victoria became a convalescence home for military officers during the First World War.
Camiers Hospital	Site of both Base and Stationary Hospitals.
Étaples	Étaples is a town about seventeen miles (twenty-seven kilometres) just south of Boulogne, in the Pas-du-Calais region of northern France. During the First World War, its environs were the scene of large concentrations of reinforcement camps and hospitals. Accessible by railway from the frontline battlefields, in 1917, 100,000 troops were camped among the sand dunes and the hospitals, which included eleven general, one stationary, four Red Cross hospitals and a convalescent depot. Étaples Military Cemetery, located to the north of the town, is the largest CWGC cemetery in France and contains 10,771 burials from the First World War, the earliest dating from May 1915. Thirty-five burials are identified.
Arras	A large town, capital of Pas-de-Calais, in the Hauts-de-France region, northern France. It lies on the Scarpe River, southwest of Lille. The Battle of Arras, also known as the Second Battle of Arras, was a British offensive on the Western Front where, from 9 April to 16 May 1917, British troops continually attacked German defences near the town. The battle became a costly stalemate for both sides, with the British suffering an estimated 160,000 casualties and the Germans around 125,000.
Hospital le Jean	A small village in the Arras region of northern France. Hospital base for the wounded. The village and hospital were all but destroyed by enemy shelling.

Warlus	Situated five miles (eight kilometres) south-west of Arras, Warlus is a district in the Somme, in northern France.
Le Treport – Base	Le Treport is a coastal town approximately nineteen miles (thirty kilometres) north-east of Dieppe. It was an important First World War hospital centre. No. 3 General Hospital was established there is November 1914; No. 16 General Hospital in February 1915; No. 2 Canadian General Hospital in March 1915; No. 3 Convalescent Depot in June 1915 and Lady Murray's BRCS Hospital in July 1916. No. 47 General Hospital arrived in March 1917 together with a divisional rest camp and tank training depot later that year. By March 1919, the hospitals had all closed and the town now became the headquarters of the 68th Division.
St Pol	The town of St Pol is eighteen miles (twenty-nine kilometres) south-west of Bethune and around twenty-one miles (thirty-four kilometres) north-west of Arras. It was a military administrative centre throughout the whole of the First World War and was taken over by Commonwealth troops from the French in March 1916. No. 12 Stationary Hospital was posted on the race-course near the town from 1 June 1916 to 1 June 1919. To the south of the town is the British War Cemetery, which has 258 Commonwealth burials, including the graves of sixteen men of the 58th Battalion AIF killed by a shell at St Pol station on 27 March 1918, and seven Australian servicemen are represented by special memorials.
la Panne	Lying on the border with France, la Panne is a town and municipality located on the North Sea coast of the Belgium province of West Flanders.

Zudycote	A small coastal town in the Nord region of northern France, approximately six miles (ten kilometres) north of Dunkirk. Throughout the First World War the local Vancauwenberghe sanatorium served as a military hospital with more than 100,000 wounded soldiers received and cared for. During the autumn of 1917, the 34th and 36th Casualty Clearing Stations were located in the town's environs. To the west of the village is the Zudycote Military Cemetery, which contains predominantly the graves of officers and men who died at the hospital, numbering 327 in total.
Passchendaele	The small village of Passchendaele lies five miles (eight kilometres) north-east of Ypres and is the name by which the Third Battle of Ypres is more commonly known by. Passchendaele became infamous not only for the scale of casualties, but also for the treacherous topography. The main battle commenced on 31 July 1917 and stretched on until 10 November 1917. Just south-west of the village is Tyne Cot, the site of the largest CWGC cemetery. 'Tyne Cot' or 'Tyne Cottage' was the name given by the Northumberland Fusiliers to a barn that once stood near the level crossing on the Passchendaele-Broodseinde Road. Some 11,961 Commonwealth servicemen buried or commemorated within the cemetery, 8,373 are unidentified. There are also four German burials, three being unidentified.
Yser-Canal	The Yser Front, sometimes termed the West Flemish Front, was a section of the Western Front during the First World War that was held by Belgians. The front line ran along the Yser river and the Yser Canal for a distance of around nineteen miles (thirty kilometres) from the Belgium Coast. The Battle of Yser took place in October 1914.

St Julien	St Julien was a village in west Flanders, north of Ypres, which lay within the Allied lines from the late autumn of 1914 until April 1915. The Germans used poison gas here for the first time on 22 April, but the village was held by 3 Canadian Infantry Brigade until a second gas attack two days later. It was recaptured by 39th Division in early August but fell into German hands again on 27 April 1918. The Belgian Army finally overran the Germans and took the village on 28 September 1918.
Arneke	The village of Arneke is located in the Nord region of northern France, thirty-one miles (fifty kilometres) south-east of Calais and about five miles (eight kilometres) north-west of Cassel. Site of Stationary Hospital throughout October 1918. Also, home to two war cemeteries. Around one mile (two kilometres) north of the village is the Arneke British War Cemetery, first constructed by 13th Casualty Clearing Station which moved to Arneke from the Proven area in October 1917. It was joined by 10th and 44th Clearing Stations in April 1918. The cemetery was used by these hospitals until the end of May, and again from July to September 1918 by 62nd (1/2nd London) Clearing Station. In November it was used for a short time by 4th and 10th Stationary Hospitals. It contains 434 Commonwealth burials, 126 French and five German war graves.
Namur (Belgium)	A fortified city located around thirty-seven miles (sixty kilometres) southeast of Brussels, today Namur is the administrative capital of so-called Wallonie, French speaking Belgium. It was the site of the Siege of Namur when, in 1914, Belgium and German forces fought around the ring-fort city.

After continual heavy shelling the city eventually fell to the Germans in August 2014.

Givenchy

A small village located in the district of Pas-de-Calais in the French region Nord-Pas-de-Calais. It became a central part of the British line and was close to the scenes of major engagements.

The Battle of Givenchy commenced in the early hours of 19 December 1914 when Indian troops from the Lahore Division launched an attack, successfully capturing two lines of German trenches. Their success was short-lived, however, and a prompt and aggressive counter-action by the Germans pushed the Indian troops back. British losses were high, especially among the Indian units.

Richbourg L'Avoue

Located in the Pas-de-Calais region of northern France. It was the site of the Battle of the Boar's Head, so named due to the peculiar boar head's shape of the network of trenches criss-crossed the salient, when on 30 June 1916 the 39th Division, XI Corps, in First Army of the British Expeditionary Force, advanced to capture the site, which was then held by the German Sixth Army.

Fromelles

Fromelles is a small village situated in the Nord/Pas de Calais region of northern France, approximately fourteen miles (twenty-two kilometres) west of Lille and sixty-four miles (104 kilometres) southeast of Calais.

Scene of one of the greatest tragedies suffered by Australian forces. The Australian 5th Division, along with 61st British (South Midland) Division, attacked here on 19 July 1916. At this time, the main Somme battles were raging around forty miles (sixty-four kilometres), to the south of Fromelles. The assault did not go to plan, with thousands of Allied men killed in a matter of minutes, the Australian Division lost 5,513 of their men in one day. British forces experienced 1,517 casualties, whilst the German forces lost between 1,600 to 2,000 men.

In 2009, archaeologists excavated several mass burial pits at Pheasant Wood near Fromelles. The remains of 250 British and Australian soldiers were recovered from these pits, which were mass burials made by the Germans after the Battle of Fromelles, and a new cemetery was subsequently created for their burial by the Commonwealth War Graves Commission, the first since the Second World War. Named Fromelles (Pheasant Wood) Cemetery, it is located at the north-west edge of the village, not far from the church and only about a quarter of a mile from Pheasant Wood itself, where the men were originally buried by the Germans. At 11 a.m. on 30 January 2010, the first of the remains were reburied at this new cemetery. Efforts to identify these men continue.

Neuve Chapelle

The operation at Neuve Chapelle in March 1915 was the first offensive conducted by the British Expeditionary Force (BEF) during the First World War. The village itself is just over three miles (five kilometres) north of la Bassée and fifteen miles (twenty kilometres) south-west of Lillle. Today, located south-west of the village is the Neuve Chapelle Memorial, which is dedicated to over 4,700 Indian soldiers and labourers who lost their lives on the Western Front and have no known graves.

Fouquieres

Fouquieres-les-Béthune is a small village, in the Pas-da-Calais region, about half a mile (one kilometre) south-west of Béthune, Hauts-du-France. The local churchyard contains 387 burials from the First World War.

Avuley Wood	Small village located just over three miles (five kilometres) north of the town of Albert. Site of Advanced Dressing Station in the Somme conflict of 1916. The British 32nd and 36th Divisions held the area from the beginning of the Battle of the Somme on 1 July 1916 to the German retreat to the Hindenburg Line in February 1917. The Germans retook the wood in April 1918 as part of a major offensive. The area was then repeatedly attacked by Allied forces until it was recaptured in August 1918. Around three miles (five kilometres) to the north of Albert, in an area known as 'Lancashire Dump,' lies Avuley Wood Cemetery. Established a few days before the Battle of the Somme, in 1916, it was continually used by fighting units and field ambulances until the withdrawal to the Hindenburg Line in 1917. It remained unused until the German advance in the spring of 1918. The cemetery contains 380 burials from the First World War, 172 are unidentified.
Contalmaison	The seventh largest village on the Somme, Contalmaison is located in the Picardy region of northern France. In 1916 the village was between the German first and second positions, each having three trenches approximately 180 metres apart. Became an area for BEF field ambulances.
Guillemont	Part of the Battle of the Somme, Guillemont is a small village that was located on the right flank of the British sector, near the boundary with the French Army. The defence of Guillemont has been judged by some observers to be the best performance of the war by the German army on the Western Front.

Talus Boise	Located in the Somme area. Known as Death Valley by forces.
Montauban-Maricourt	The village of Montauban lay behind the German frontline, and had been heavily fortified, whilst the town of Maricourt lay behind British lines of defence. Both are located in the Somme valley, in the Picardy and Hauts-de-France regions of northern France. On the first day of the Battle of the Somme, July 1916, military operations commenced with heavy fighting and the attempted capture of Montauban, with heavy casualties borne by both sides. Maricourt was later lost in the German advance of March 1918 but recaptured the following August. The Montauban-Maricourt areas contain a number of war cemeteries. For example, to the west of Maricourt village there sits Peronne Road Cemetery, previously known as Maricourt Military Cemetery No. 3, begun by fighting units and field ambulances at the Battle of the Somme in 1916. It was in constant use until August 1917. At the Armistice it consisted of 175 burials. To the south of the village there lies Maricourt French Military Cemetery, which contains the burial of one British soldier.

Appendix IV

Base Hospitals on the Western Front

The following list documents both General and Stationary hospitals that operated from the outset of the war to after the Armistice.

Abbeville	No. 3 British Red Cross, Oct 14-Jan 16
Aire	No. 39 Stationary. May 17-Jly 18
Amiens	No. 7 General, Aug – Sep 14; No. 1 New Zealand Stationary. Jly 16 – May 17; No. 41 Stationary. Mar 18 – Jan 19; No. 42 Stationary. Oct 17 – Apr
Angiens	No 5 General Sep 15 – Feb 15
Antwerp	No 6 Stationary from Apr 19 onwards
Arneke	No 10 Stationary Oct 18
Arques	No 4 Stationary May 18 – Nov 18
Bonn	No 47 General Apr 19 onwards
Boulogne	No 7 British Red Cross Oct 14 – Jan 15; No 7 General May 18 – Apr 19; No 7 Stationary Oct 14 – Apr 19; No 8 British Red Cross Jan 18 onwards; No 11 General Oct 14 – Apr 16; No 13 General Oct 14 – Feb 19; No 13 Stationary Oct 14 – Jun 16; No 14 Stationary Jun 19 – Jan 20; No 83 General Jun 16 – Apr 19
Bruges	Military Hospital Nov 18 – Jan 19
Calais	No 8 British Red Cross Oct 14 – Jly 15; No 9 British Red Cross Jan 16 – Mar 18; No 35 General May 15 – Dec 19; No 38 Stationary Jly 17 – Nov 17; Isolation Hospital Dec 15 – Dec 18; No 2 Anglo-Belgium BRCS Hospital Apr 15 – Dec 19
Camiers	No 4 General Jan 16 – Apr 19; No 11 General Apr 16 – May 17; No 18 General Feb 15 – Jun 17;

	No 20 General May 15 – Apr 19; No 22 General Jun 15 – Jan 19; No 42 Stationary Apr 18 – Nov 18
Charmes	Detention Hospital Mar 19 onwards
Clerques	No 10 Stationary Jun 18 – Oct 18
Dannes-Camiers	No 25 General Aug 15 – May 16
Desvres	No 39 Stationary Jly 18 – Aug 18
Dieppe	No 5 British Red Cross A Section Jan 15 – May 19; Detention Hospital Apr 17 onwards
Dunkirk	No 4 General Apr 19 – Nov 19
Duren	No 11 Stationary Mar 19 onwards
Étaples	No 6 British Red Cross Jly 15 – Jun 18; No 7 British Red Cross Aug 15 – Nov 15; No 23 General Jun 15 – Nov 16; No 24 General Jun 15 – Jly 19; No 46 Stationary Jly 15 – Jun 19; No 51 General (VD) Oct 16 – Oct 19; No 56 General Mar 17 – Apr 19; St Johns Ambulance Brigade Hospital Jly 15 – Jly18
Etretat	No 1 General Dec 14 – Jan 19
Euskirchan	No 42 Stationary May 19 onward
Fillievres	No 6 Stationary Sep 18 – Feb 19
Forges-les-Eaux	BRCS Detention Hospital Apr 15 – Apr 19
Fort Gassin	No 39 Stationary Sep 18 – Apr 19
Fouilloy	No 41 Stationary Apr 18
Frevent	No 6 Stationary Jun 16 – Aug 18
Gailly	No 41 Stationary May 17 – Mar 18
Gournay-en-Bray	BRCS Detention Hospital Feb 15 – Apr 19
Hardelot	No 25 General Jun 16 – Jly 17
Harfleur	No 40 Stationary May 17 – Nov 19
Hazebrouck	No 1 New Zealand Stationary May 17 – Sep 17; No 9 British Red Cross Sep 18 – Oct 18
le Havre	No 1 General Aug 14 – Nov 14; No 2 General Aug 14 – May 19; No 6 Stationary Dec 14 – May 16; No 9 Stationary Aug-Sep 14 & Oct 14; No 39 General Jun 16; No 25 Stationary Oct 15 – Jly 19
Hesdin	Detention Hospital Jan 19 – Feb 19
Langenfeld	No 83 General Apr 19 onwards
le Mans	No 1 Stationary Sep 14 – Oct 14; No 5 Stationary Sep 15 – Dec 14; No 10 Stationary Sep 14 – Oct 14

le Touquet   No 1 British Red Cross Oct 14 – Jly 18

le Treport   No 3 General Nov 14 – Mar 19; No 10 British Red Cross Jun 16 – Dec 18; No 16 General Jan 15 – Feb 19; No 47 General Apr 17 – Mar 19

Longuenesse   No 4 Stationary Dec 18 onwards; No 9 British Red Cross Mar 18 – Aug 18

Marseilles   Rawalpindi British General Oct 14 – Dec 14; Lahore British General Jan 15 – Apr 15; Marseilles Stationary Aug 16 – Mar 19; Section of No 39 General Hospital present from Jun 16; No 57 General Jly 17 – Feb 20; No 81 General Dec 17 – Apr 19

Nancy   No 42 Stationary Nov 18 – Mar 19

Nantes   No 2 Stationary Sep 14 – Nov 14; No 9 General Sep 14 – Nov 14

Orlcans   No 10 Stationary briefly active in Oct 14; Meerut British General Oct 14 – Dec 14

Outreau   No 2 Stationary Nov 14 – Sep 15

Paris   Detention Hospital Aug 16 onwards; Stationary Hospital Jun 18 – May 19

Paris-Plage   No 6 British Red Cross Apr 15 – Jly 15; No 8 British Red Cross Sep 15 – Dec 17

Poulainville   No 41 Stationary Feb 19 – Nov 19

Pont Remy   No 41 Stationary Apr 18 – Nov 18

Remy Siding   No 10 Stationary Feb 19 onwards

Rotterdam   No 3 Stationary Apr 19 onwards

Roubaix   No 9 British Red Cross Oct 18 – Nov 18

Rouderbirken   No 3 General Mar 19 onwards

Rouen   No 1 Stationary Oct 14 (?); No 2 British Red Cross Sep 14 – Dec 18 (?); No 3 General Aug 14 – Sep 14; No 3 Stationary Feb 15 – Mar 19; No 5 general Aug 14 – Sep 14 & Feb 15 – Mar 19; No 6 General Nov 14 – Apr 19; No 8 General Aug 14 – May 19; No 9 General Nov 14 – Jun 17; No 10 General Oct 14 – May 19; No 11 Stationary Oct 14 – Mar 19; No 12 General Sep 14 – Jun 17; No 12 Stationary Feb 15 – May 16; No 25 Stationary Mar 15 – May 19; No 58 General Apr 18 – Mar 19; No 59 General Apr

	18 – Mar 19; Meerut British General Jan 15 – Aug 15; No 2 Australian General
St Nazaire	Australian Voluntary Hospital Sep – Oct 14; No 3 General Sep 14 – Nov 14; No 4 General Sep 14; No 9 Stationary Sep 14 – Oct 14; No 10 General Sep 14 – Oct 14; No 32 Stationary Sep 14 – Jly 16
St Omer	No 4 Stationary 14 – 18; No 7 General Jun 15 – May 18; No 10 Stationary Oct 14 – May 18; No 58 General Aug 17 – Mar 18; No 59 General Jly 17 – Mar 18
St Pol	No 12 Stationary Jun 16 – Jun 19
Tourcoing	No 10 Stationary Nov 18 – Feb 19
Trouville	No 6 British Red Cross Sep 18 – Dec 18; No 72 General Dec 17 – Oct 19; No 73 General Feb 18 – Apr 19; No 74 General Mar 18 – Mar 19; St Johns Ambulance Brigade Hospital from Jly 18
Versailles	No 4 General Sep 14 – Jan 16
Wisedorf	No 25 General Mar 19 onwards
Wimereux	Australian Voluntary Hospital Oct 14 – Jly 16; No 4 British Red Cross Nov 14 – Dec 15; No 5 British Red Cross Dec 14 – Jan 19; No 8 Stationary Mar 15 – Mar 19; No 14 General Oct 14 – Apr 19; No 14 Stationary Oct 14 – Jun; No 32 Stationary Jly 16 – Dec 19; No 54 General Jly 17 – May 19; No 32 Stationary Jly 16 – Dec 19; No 54 General Jly 17 – May 19; No 53 General Jly 17 – Feb 19; No 55 General May 17 – Mar 19; BRCS Auxiliary Hospital Dec 15 – Mar 19; Rawalpindi British General Jan 15
Wisques	No 1 New Zealand Stationary Sep 1917 onwards

Appendix V

Classification of wounds used by British Army

The following classification of wounds appears in the few admissions registers that remain from the conflict and are held at the National Archives in Kew (collection MH106). They are sometimes seen in the notes recording wounds on a man's service record.

1. **Gunshot wounds of the head**
   - Contusions and simple flesh wounds of the scalp
   - With fracture of the cranium without depression
   - With fracture of the cranium with depression
   - Penetrating the cranium
   - Perforating the cranium
2. **Gunshot wounds of the face**
   - Simple flesh contusions and wounds
   - With fracture
   - Fracture with lesion
   - With fracture of the lower jaw
3. **Gunshot wounds of the neck**
   - Simple flesh contusions and wounds
   - With injury of the ...
4. **Gunshot wounds of the chest**
   - Simple flesh contusions and wounds
   - With injury of bony or cartilaginous parietes without lesion of contents
   - With lesion of contents by contusion, or with non-penetrating wound
   - Penetrating
   - Implicating contents

5. **Gunshot wounds of the abdomen**
   - Simple flesh contusions and wounds
   - Contusion or non-penetrating wound with lesion of …
   - Penetrating or perforating, with lesion of …
6. **Gunshot wounds of the back and spine**
   - Simple flesh contusions and wounds
   - With fracture of vertebra, without lesion of spinal cord
   - With fracture and lesion of spinal cord
7. **Gunshot contusions and wounds of the perineum and genital urinary organs, not being at the same time wounds of the peritoneum**
8. **Gunshot wounds of the upper extremities**
   - Simple flesh contusions and wounds
   - With contusion or fracture of long bones
   - Simple fracture of long bones by contusion
   - Compound fracture of …
9. **Gunshot wounds of the lower extremities**
   - Simple flesh contusions and wounds
   - With contusion or fracture of long bones
   - Simple fracture of long bones by contusion
   - Compound fracture of …
10. **Gunshot wounds with direct injury of the large arteries not being at the same time cases of compound fracture**
11. **Gunshot wounds with direct penetration or perforation of the larger joints**
12. **Gunshot wounds with direct injury of the large nerves not being at the same time cases of compound fracture**
13. **Wounds caused by sword or lance**
14. **Bayonet wounds**
15. **Miscellaneous wounds**

Appendix VI

Trench Foot and Lice

If life on the Western Front was not challenging enough, during the course of the war the human foot would experience continual anguish and torment. The problem being that in France, and particularly throughout Flanders, the field of conflict was often found to be at, or near to, sea level, or the water table lay just beneath the soil surface. Therefore, as the soldiers began to burrow down into the soil, after only a few feet of excavation they would inevitably hit the water table, causing the trenches to flood. Heavy shelling by the Germans also contributed to the matter, as their continual barrages of artillery would destroy the surrounding agricultural land drains, transforming the landscape into a sea of mud. In fact, the trenches became so wet that in one sector German soldiers reportedly began sitting on top of the trench walls just to dry off. British soldiers soon followed suit, shouting 'don't shoot' at their counterparts, until an order came through from GHQ that such 'fraternisation' would not be tolerated.

Trench Foot first appeared during the winter of 1914-15 when it became apparent that a new debilitating condition was troubling the men in ever-increasing numbers. Characterised by swelling and pain, the feet of those afflicted would gradually go numb, the skin turning an intense colour of red or blue. In rare cases the feet could also become gangrenous and would thus require amputation. Quickly recognised by the military authorities, and, after much deliberation with various names, the term 'trench foot' was officially endorsed by the War Office, despite the DMS First Army noting that:

> (the) term Trench feet is to be discontinued and 'chilled feet' substituted, it seems to me that the terms 'Trench' feet, 'Trench' fever etc are likely to centre too much attention on

the trench inconveniences in the soldier's mind and he is
too much on the look-out for diseases caused or said to be
caused by being in the trenches.

By the end of that particular winter, over 20,000 British soldiers had
received treatment for trench foot. Remedies involved a number of
conventional, tried-and-tested, methods, some working better than others,
with medical officers often left to their own devices in experimenting
with different cures. These included putting rum in boots, which proved
useless; and the placing of braziers of burning charcoal in the trenches,
but this did more harm than good. Moreover, wrapping the infected feet
in cotton wool appeared to aggravate the condition. Ultimately, soldiers
were ordered to dry their feet continually, change their socks several
times a day, and cover their feet with a grease-like concoction made
from whale oil, after which, on no account were they to be held in front
of a fire! It has been estimated that a battalion on the front line would use
up to ten gallons of whale oil every day. Some units even implemented
a 'stamping drill,' whereby the men would stomp and rub their feet in
unison to get the blood flow going.

Further practical measures included the digging of draining ditches
in the trenches, to alleviate the water flow, as well as the placement
of duckboards, initially introduced by the 1st Battalion Royal Irish
Fusiliers, between communication trenches, to avoid flooding. New
time limits were imposed on the men, whereby soldiers were limited
to thirty-six hours spent in a waterlogged trench at any given time,
whilst the importance of maintaining comfortable, warm waterproof
boots was stressed. Research into the ailment continued throughout the
war, coupled with the availability of new innovative treatments, such as
socks prepared with borax, invented by Scottish engineer John Logie
Baird, inventor of the TV system. These became extremely popular
and were widely used by soldiers at the front. But the principal factor
in the disease's prevention was the skill of the MO in recognising the
situation before it 'got out of hand'. It was the MO's responsibility to
keep a regular check on the men's feet, and to ensure that combatant
officers remained attentive to this important matter bearing upon the
fighting efficiency of the men. Even so, by the end of the war around
75,000 Allied troops had been affected by the condition. One, officer,

Brigadier General Frank Percy Crozier was quoted as saying 'the fight against the condition known as trench-feet had been incessant and an uphill game'.

An additional problem, rife throughout the trenches, which gave the military authorities a perpetual headache, was the existence of lice. Commonly referred to as 'chats,' these tiny insects would hide in the seams of soldiers' clothes, leaving blotchy red bite marks all over their bodies. Pale beige in colour, their reproduction cycle was prolific, with each female capable of producing as many as a dozen fresh eggs per day, which could hatch within a month. A requirement for the insect's survival was warm, moist conditions, so the cramped surroundings of trench warfare were the ideal environment for them, particularly as the newly-hatched offspring were in close proximity to a new host. For the men, it was torment, especially as they would only be offered a full bath two or three times per month. It is estimated that up to 97 per cent of officers and men who worked and lived in the trenches were afflicted with lice at one time or another.

Apart from the skin irritation lice would convey, they also carried a disease known as 'trench fever' which could incapacitate a soldier for months at a time. Understandably, this put enormous pressure on the medical authorities because not only were the infected not able to fight, but they also appropriated much needed hospital beds. On average the casualty rate attributed to trench fever hovered around fifteen per cent. First reported in mid-1915 by physicians of the BEF on the Western Front, within a few short months hundreds of cases had been clinically identified. Highly infectious, trench fever is characterised by a sudden onset of fever, headache, pain behind the eyes, weakness, sore muscles and joints, and often severe pain in the back and shins. Initially, the military believed that the illness was nothing more than an infection, on similar lines to that of malaria, as a reported increase of cases in the summer combined with a decreasing caseload in winter gave credence to the diagnosis of a mosquito-borne organism. However, by 1916, it was generally agreed that the louse was the most likely culprit and, by 1917, a year before the end of the war, the War Office officially designated the disease Trench Fever.

The treatment of Trench Fever throughout the First World War was pretty much hit and miss. Every pharmaceutical treatment thought to have promise was tried without much success, although the British did have some success with a paste combining naphthalene, creosote and iodine, which the men could apply to the seams of their uniforms, killing any lice present in only a few hours. Another favoured method employed by the men was to run a candle, or cigarette, along the seams of clothing, which the insect would typically inhabit. They would often gather in groups to have, what they called, 'a chat,' namely a group de-lousing session whereby the lice would be sought, found and then crushed between their fingernails. By the end of war, it is estimated that the total number of cases of Trench Fever among troops on the Western Front reached almost 500,000.

Appendix VII

A Brief History of
The Lancashire Fusiliers

The Lancashire Fusiliers was a line infantry battalion of the British Army that served many years of distinguished service. Originally formed in 1688, in Devon, as Peyton's Regiment of Foot, so named after the commanding colonel Sir Richard Peyton, it was active during the early days of the Jacobite Rebellion, when the regiment helped defeat King James II's forces at the Battle of the Boyne in 1690 as well as playing a crucial role at Aughrim in 1691.

The regiment went on to serve in the War of the Spanish Succession (1701-14) and the War of the Austrian Succession, distinguishing itself at the Battles of Dettingen (1743) and Fontenoy (1745). During yet another Jacobite Rebellion, when Bonnie Prince Charlie (grandson of James II) tried to claim the throne instead of the Hanoverian King George I, the regiment also served at the Battle of Culloden. In 1751 the tradition of changing the regiment's name to that of the commanding colonel was replaced with ranked numbers of precedence and the regiment became known thereafter as the 20th Regiment of Foot.

In 1752 James Wolfe (later the famous General Wolfe) joined the regiment as lieutenant colonel and fought with it during the Seven Years' War (1754-1763) until 1758. At the Battle of Minden in 1759, the regiment distinguished itself when the infantry formation broke the French cavalry charge. The regiment was also involved in the American Revolutionary War (1775-83) and was sent to Quebec in 1776 to assist in the city's siege and capture from the French, fighting once again under the command of General James Wolfe until his death. However, the regiment was later forced to surrender to the American army at Saratoga along with 5,800 men, when General John Burgoyne surrendered his entire army during a campaign to capture New York.

In 1782 all British regiments without Royal titles were awarded county titles in order to aid recruitment and the regiment became the 20th (East Devonshire) Regiment. It went onto serve during the Crimean War (1853-56) fighting at the Alma and Inkerman and in the first Sudan War (1884-85). In 1881 the Childers Reforms restructured the British army infantry into a network of multi-battalion contingents, at first the regiment maintained their XXth nomenclature, but soon the number of precedence was dropped and thus the regiment became known as the Lancashire Fusiliers. The regiment went on to serve during the Second Boer War (1899-1902), fighting at Spion Kop and the Relief of Ladysmith in 1900.

At the beginning of 1915, the Lancashire Fusiliers were active in Karachi, India, soon returning home to Britain at the end of January. With the First World War intensifying, in April 1915, the battalion made its way to Gallipoli, as part of 86 Brigade in 29th Division, landing at Cape Helles under heavy gunfire. Here the Regiment earned six Victoria Crosses, the landing spot (W Beach) becoming known as 'Lancashire Landing'. The battalion was evacuated in January 1916 and diverted to Marseille, France in March 1916 where they first saw action on the Western Front. In total the regiment raised thirty battalions during the First World War and was awarded sixty-three Battle Honours and six Victoria Crosses, losing 13,640 men during the course of the war. In honour of the lives sacrificed during the Great War, a memorial to the regiment, commissioned in honour of its First World War casualties, was erected outside Wellington Barracks in Bury, opposite the regimental headquarters. It was designed by Sir Edwin Lutyens, famous for the Cenotaph in London, whose father and great uncle served in the Lancashire Fusiliers. With the later demolition of the barracks, the memorial was relocated to Gallipoli Garden in the town.

With the reduction in regiments to a single regular battalion, a process that commenced in 1947, together with the withdrawal of troops from India and other Commonwealth counties, as well as the decision to have no forces east of Suez, bar the Hong Kong garrison, on 23 April 1968, the regiment was merged with the Royal Northumberland Fusiliers, The Royal Warwickshire Fusiliers and The Royal Fusiliers (City of London

Regiment) to form The Royal Regiment of Fusiliers of the Queen's Division. Now consisting of one regular and one Army Reserve battalion, the Fusiliers have seen service across the world and found themselves at the sharp end in regions as diverse as Northern Ireland and Cyprus. More recently the Regiment served in Kosovo and the Balkans, took part in both the First and Second Gulf Wars and did several operational tours in Afghanistan.

Appendix VIII

A Brief History of
The Manchester Regiment

For a period of approximately twenty years, from the 1860s to the 1880s, the British Army underwent a period of reforms, whereby single-battalion regiments were amalgamated and affiliated under a geographical area. Known as the Childers Reforms, so named after Hugh Childers and Edward Cardwell, the Manchester Regiment, a line infantry regiment was created on 1 July 1881 by the joining of the 63rd (West Suffolk) Regiment of Foot and the 96th Regiment of Foot as the 1st and 2nd Battalions. The latter had been raised in the town of Manchester in 1824. Eight additional battalions were gained through the incorporation of the 6th Royal Lancashire Militia and rifle corps units from Lancashire. By July, the regiment had the following under its command:

- Regimental Headquarters
- 63rd Regimental District (Regimental Depot) based in Ashton (later named Ladysmith Barracks)
- 1st Battalion (Regular)
- 2nd Battalion (Regular)
- 3rd (1st Battalion, 6th Royal Lancashire Militia) Battalion (Militia)
- 4th (2nd Battalion, 6th Royal Lancashire Militia) Battalion (Militia)
- 1st Volunteer Battalion – former 4th Lancashire Rifle Volunteers
- 2nd Volunteer Battalion – former 6th Lancashire (1st Manchester) Rifle Volunteers
- 3rd Volunteer Battalion – former 40th Lancashire (3rd Manchester) Rifle Volunteers
- 4th Volunteer Battalion – former 20th Lancashire (2nd Manchester) Rifle Volunteers

- 5th (Ardwick) Volunteer Battalion – former 23rd Lancashire Rifle Volunteers
- 6th Volunteer Battalion – former 7th Lancashire Rifle Volunteers

In 1882, both the 1st and 2nd Battalions saw action against Urabi Pasha's revolt in Egypt, they also undertook garrison duties at various locations around the British Empire, such as India, Malta, and Aden. In 1897, the 2nd Battalion also served on the North West Frontier to quell a tribal uprising. In 1899 the 1st Battalion was deployed to fight in the Second Boer War (1899-1902) where it saw action at Elandslaagte (1899) and the defence of Ladysmith (1899) respectively. At that time, the 2nd Battalion was stationed in Ireland, but relieved the 1st Battalion in South Africa in 1900, located in the Orange Free State. During the Boer War the regiment raised two more regular battalions, the 3rd and 4th, the former stationed on St Helena and South Africa, whilst the latter remained in Ireland. Both battalions were disbanded in 1906.

At the outbreak of the First World War in August 1914, the 2nd Battalion, who were stationed in the UK, were deployed to France immediately, as part of the 5th Division, and stayed on the Western Front throughout the conflict. Having supported the Expeditionary Force's retreat following the Battle of Mons, they were soon engaged in the battles of the Marne, the Aisne and First Ypres. Whereas the 1st Battalion, who were stationed in India, left for France with haste, as part of the Indian Expeditionary Force, arriving in Marseille in September of that year. Briefly attached to the French Cavalry, the 1st Battalion moved to the front line on 26 October, relieving a battalion of the Bedfordshire Regiment at Festubert. It served on the Western Front until December 1915, when it moved to Mesopotamia for two years, later transferring to Egypt in April 1918 and then Palestine two months later.

On 1 July 1916, the regiment had nine battalions on the Front, including the Manchester Pals, the 16th (1st City), 17th (2nd City), 18th (3rd City) and 19th (4th City), all serving in 90 Brigade of 30th Division. Sadly, this day proved to be the deadliest in the British Army's history, with almost 20,000 men killed in action. Nevertheless, the regiment continued its involvement in the Somme Offensive. For example, in late July the 16th, 17th and 18th Manchesters attacked an area in the vicinity of the small village of Guillemont. During the action, Company

Sergeant Major George Evans, of the 18th, volunteered to deliver an important message, having witnessed five previous fatal attempts to do so. He delivered his message, running more than half a mile despite being wounded. He was awarded the Victoria Cross. On 2 April 1917 the 2nd Manchesters attacked Francilly-Selency, in which C Company captured a battery of 77mm guns and a number of machine guns, whilst later in the month, the Manchester Regiment fought in the Arras Offensive. During the Third Battle of Ypres, more commonly referred to as Passchendaele, the Manchester Pals' Brigade fought in the offensive's opening battle, at Pilckem Ridge, on 31 July. The regiment also raised nineteen Territorial and sixteen New Army battalions for various theatres of conflict, some of which served at Gallipoli in 1915 and Salonika in 1915-1918, whilst others fought in France and Flanders and at home stations.

After serving on the Western Front from July 1915 the 12th (Service) Battalion amalgamated with the Regimental HQ and two squadrons of the Manchester-based Duke of Lancaster's Own Yeomanry (DLOY), who had been dismounted and retrained as infantry. From 24 September 1917 the battalion was redesignated the 12th (DLOY) Battalion, Manchester Regiment. It continued serving with 17th (Northern Division until the Armistice, seeing action at the Battle of Passchendaele, and the German Spring Offensive of 1918

The English poet Wilfred Owen served with the 2nd Battalion Manchesters in the later stages of the war. On 1 October 1918 he led various elements of the battalion in the raid of enemy strongpoints near the village of Joncourt. For his courage and leadership in the Joncourt action, he was awarded the Military Cross. He was killed in action, on 4 November 1918, during the crossing of the Sambre-Oise Canal, exactly one week (almost to the hour) before the signing of the Armistice of 11 November 1918. He was promoted to the rank of lieutenant the day after his death.

After the war, in 1919, the 2nd Battalion moved to India for a year, followed by two years in Iraq. It then returned to India until it deployed to the Sudan in 1932. Meanwhile, the Manchesters returned to Britain for a year, before reinforcing the garrison in Ireland, which saw action during the Irish War of Independence (1919-21), before serving as occupation troops in Germany during the 1920s. It returned to Britain in 1927 and, in 1933, departed for the West Indies. After being posted to Egypt in

1936, the 1st Manchesters shifted into a machine-gun battalion, as did the Royal Northumberland Fusiliers, the Cheshire Regiment and the Middlesex, which also included Princess Louise's Kensington Regiment. At once they were deployed to the Mandate of Palestine where elements of the populace had begun to rebel against British authority. In 1937 a company on detachment in Cyprus provided a special guard for the Coronation parade. In 1938 the battalion moved to Singapore.

With the outbreak of the Second World War, in 1939, the 2nd Battalion, which was stationed in Britain, deployed to France. Together with the 5th and the 1/9th Manchesters they formed part of the British Expeditionary Force, who were later forced to evacuate from a number of ports sited along the French coast. They remained in Britain, recovering from their exploits, until June 1942, when the battalion was sent to India, then Burma, seeing action at Imphal-Kohima in 1944. Meanwhile the 1st Battalion Manchesters was deployed to Singapore in 1938, as part of 2 Malaya Infantry Brigade, and saw action during the Japanese invasion of the island in February 1942. After a bitter defence, Lieutenant General Arthur Percival signed the surrender of Singapore on 15 February. A few months later, in May, the regiment's 6th Battalion was renamed the 1st Battalion to replace it. This new 1st Battalion remained in Britain until 1944 when it was shipped to Normandy. It fought at Caen and Falaise, later fighting its way across north-west Europe, reaching Hamburg by the end of the war. Two of the regiment's Territorial battalions, namely 1/9th and 5th, also fought in France during 1940. The 7th fought throughout North-West Europe, whilst the 8th and 9th Battalions served in Italy, for which the regiment received eight battle honours.

The 1st Battalion's post-war role was as part of the British Army of the Rhine (BAOR) occupation of Germany until it returned to Britain in 1947. Here it was joined by the 2nd Battalion where, in 1948, the two battalions were amalgamated. With the exception of two years' service during the Malayan Emergency, from 1951 the regiment remained in Germany with the British Army of the Rhine. In 1958 the Manchester Regiment was amalgamated with The King's Regiment (Liverpool) to form The King's Regiment; the sub-title Manchester and Liverpool was dropped in 1968. Today, it is part of the Duke of Lancaster's Regiment.

Notes and References

The following textual accounts and online resources were invaluable during the research process of this book and have been utilised during the course of the supplementary text to provide an in-depth overview to the subject matter.

Textual Sources

Blair, John S.G., *In Arduis Fidelis: Centenary History of the Royal Army Medical Corps* (Edinburgh: Scottish Academic Press, 1998)

Gray, H.M.W., *The Early Treatment of War Wounds* (London: Joint Committee of Henry Frowde and Hodder & Stoughton, 1919).

McLaughlin, Redmond, *The Royal Army Medical Corps* (London: Leo Cooper Ltd, 1972).

Meyer, Jessica, *An Equal Burden: The Men of the Royal Medical Corps in the First World War*, Oxford University Press, 2019.

Royal Army Medical Corps Training (London: His Majesty's Stationery Office, 1911; repr. 1915).

Vivian, Charles, *With the Royal Army Medical Corps (RAMC) at the Front* (London: Hodder & Stoughton, 1914). War Office,

Royal Army Medical Corps Training (London: His Majesty's Stationery Office, 1911; repr. 1915).

Whitehead, Ian R., *Doctors in the Great War* (London: Leo Cooper, 1999).

Museums and Archives

The National Archives – www.nationalarchives.gov.uk
The Imperial War Museum – www.iwm.org.uk

The Wellcome Collection – www.wellcomecollection.org
The British Library – www.bl.uk
The National Library of Scotland – www.nls.uk
Lancashire Fusiliers Museum – www.fusiliermuseum.com
Manchester Regiment – www.tameside.gov.uk/archives/manchesterregiment
The Liddle Collection – www.leeds.ac.uk
Online Reference - www.jstor.org
Online Reference - www.archive.org

Online References

The Western Front Association – www.westernfrontassociation.com
The Long, Long Trail – www.longlongtrail.co.uk
RAMC in the Great War – www.ramc-ww1.com
International Encyclopaedia of First World War – www.encycopedia.1914-1918-online.net
US WW1 Centennial Commission – www.worldwar1centennial.org
A multi-media history of WW1 – www.firstworldwar.com
History Hit – www.historyhit.com
Maritime Archaeology Trust – www.forgottonwrecks.org

Select Bibliography

Arthur, Max, *Forgotten Voices of the Great War*, Ebury Press, 2003.

Blair, John S.G., *In Arduis Fidelis: Centenary History of the Royal Army Medical Corps* Edinburgh: Scottish Academic Press, 1998.

Falls, Cyril, *British Official History of Military Operations, France and Flanders*, Vol. 1, 1917.

Farr, Don., *A Battle Too Far*, Helion and Company, 2018

Fitzharris, L., *The Facemaker: One Surgeon's Battle to Mend the Disfigured Soldiers of World War I*, Allen Lane, 2022.

Gilbert, M., *Somme: The Heroism and Horror of War*, John Murray Press, 2007

Gray, H.M.W., *The Early Treatment of War Wounds*, London: Joint Committee of Henry Frowde and Hodder & Stoughton, 1919.

Gray, H.M.W. and K.M. Walker, *The Treatment of Wounded Men in Regimental Aid Posts and Field Ambulances* (Third Field Survey Company, 1916)

Herrick, Claire E.J. *Casualty Care during the First World War: The Experience of the Royal Navy. War in History* Vol. 7 No. 2 April 2000, pp. 154-179.

Holts, Major & Mrs, *Concise Illustrated Battlefield Guide to The Western Front – North*, Pen and Sword Military, 2004

Horton, Charles H., *Stretcher-Bearer: Fighting for Life in the Trenches*, Lion Books, 2013

Gordon, Huntly, *The Unreturning Army*, Bantam Press, 2015.

Kendall, Paul, *The Battle of Neuve Chapelle: Britain's Forgotten Offensive 1915*, Frontline Books, 2016.

Levine, Joseph, *Forgotten Voices of the Somme*, Ebury Press, 2009

Liddle, Peter, *Passchendaele in Perspective: The Third Battle of Ypres*, Pen and Sword, 1998

MacDonald, Lyn, *The Roses of No Man's Land*, Penguin Books, 2013.

_____, *They Call It Passchendaele*, Penguin Books, 1993

McLaughlin, Redmond, *The Royal Army Medical Corps* London: Leo Cooper Ltd, 1972.

Meyer, Jessica, *An Equal Burden: The Men of the Royal Medical Corps in the First World War*, Oxford University Press, 2019.

Royal Army Medical Corps Training (London: His Majesty's Stationery Office, 1911; repr. 1915).

Steel, N. & Hart P., *Passchendaele: The Sacrificial Ground*, Cassell Military Paperbacks, Orion Publishing Group, 2001

Stevenson, David, *1914-1918: The History of the First World War*, Penguin, 2012.

Stewart A., & Stewart A. Captain, *A Very Unimportant Officer: Life and Death on the Somme and at Passchendaele*, Hodder and Stoughton, 2009

Vivian, Charles, *With the Royal Army Medical Corps (R.A.M.C.) at the Front*, London: Hodder & Stoughton, 1914, War Office.

Whitehead, Ian R., *Doctors in the Great War*, London, Leo Cooper, 1999.